LGBTQ+ PEOPLE and DEMENTIA

A Good Practice Guide

Sue Westwood and
Elizabeth Price

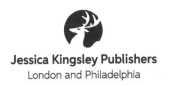

Jessica Kingsley Publishers
London and Philadelphia

First published in Great Britain in 2023 by Jessica Kingsley Publishers
An imprint of John Murray Press

2

Copyright © Sue Westwood and Elizabeth Price 2023

The right of Sue Westwood and Elizabeth Price to be identified as
the Author of the Work has been asserted by them in accordance
with the Copyright, Designs and Patents Act 1988.

A CIP catalogue record for this title is available from
the British Library and the Library of Congress

ISBN 978 1 83997 330 7
eISBN 978 1 83997 331 4

Printed and bound in the United States by Integrated Books International

Jessica Kingsley Publishers' policy is to use papers that are natural,
renewable and recyclable products and made from wood grown in
sustainable forests. The logging and manufacturing processes are expected
to conform to the environmental regulations of the country of origin.

Jessica Kingsley Publishers
Carmelite House
50 Victoria Embankment
London EC4Y 0DZ

www.jkp.com

John Murray Press
Part of Hodder & Stoughton Limited
An Hachette UK Company

Contents

Acknowledgments

Many thanks to friends and colleagues who have very kindly supported this project, often with their own thoughts, comments and insights from their personal experiences. Special thanks go to: Kathryn Almack, Terri Clark, Tim Johnston, Rebecca Jones and Andrew Yip. We appreciate Sally Knocker's comments on an early draft of Chapter 1.

Our thanks too to those authors and organizations whose work we have cited, and, where we have quoted them extensively, given us their permission to do so.

Introduction

Chapter summary

This chapter:

✓ explains why this book is needed

✓ outlines how the book is structured and how it can be used

✓ defines and explains key terms

✓ discusses the differences between LGBTQ+ people

✓ provides a timeline and explanation of LGBTQ+ histories

✓ explores the key issues relating to LGBTQ+ people and dementia care, and the implications for dementia service providers

✓ ends with a 'Food for thought' section, to encourage ongoing reflection, discussion and debate.

Introduction

Why a good practice guide about lesbian, gay, bisexual, trans, queer plus (LGBTQ+) people affected by dementia?

I'm finding hospitals and things like that overwhelming. I'm vulnerable sometimes, not being able to fight my corner... And I wonder who is going to advocate for me when I am in that position. I am going to have to depend on other people. And I want those people I depend on to recognize my difference and acknowledge what that might mean to me. *Diana, lesbian, aged 69* (Westwood, 2016b, p.1500)

Sometimes health and social care staff say that they do not understand why LGBTQ+ people with dementia should be treated any differently from other people with dementia. They say 'we treat everyone the same' (Simpson, Almack & Walthery, 2018). The trouble is, sometimes equality is not about treating everyone the same. It is about *treating everyone differently*, according to their own needs, in order to ensure that they receive the *same quality care*.

When Clive, in his 70s, came out to the carers supporting his partner who had dementia, the carers replied that they treated everybody the same. While the response sought to reassure Clive, it also led him to question how far service providers truly consider the specific support needs and sexual identities of LGBT people. Clive said: 'We immediately said, "That's not what we want. We don't want to be treated the same...we want to be treated as a gay couple."' (National Care Forum, 2016, p.9)[1]

LGBTQ+ people with dementia may have experienced prejudice and discrimination across their lives. Particularly given that, at present at least, they are likely to be from a generation that has experienced greater hostility and prejudice than is the case for the general population. This inevitably affects how they feel about health and social care services, and, in particular, they fear that they may face further prejudice and discrimination at a time when they are especially vulnerable because of dementia.

LGBTQ+ people 'want to feel safe and be free from discrimination whether from people providing, services, other people using services or from the wider community'. (Baker & Maegusuku-Hewett, 2011, p.32)

---

1   The National Care Forum has asked us to note that since the production of this publication, there has been significant development and enhanced practice by providers.

They are also worried that care providers will not be aware of their histories and cultures, and will not recognize or support the relationships that are important to them. Sometimes this means LGBTQ+ people avoid care and support even when they badly need it.

> I would like carers not to think I am gay if my partner is a man, or straight if my partner is a woman. I am bisexual, whoever my partner is. (Anonymous)

It is important that care providers are not only equipped to respond to the needs of LGBTQ+ people living with dementia, but that they are able to demonstrate this from the outset, to allay the fears and concerns these people have about needing care, especially dementia care.

We think you will agree, there is nothing exceptional, or particularly special, here. LGBTQ+ people want to be treated as individuals who may have different experiences and lifestyles from the people who are supporting and caring from them (and from each other!), but what lies at the heart of what they want and expect is respect, validation, acceptance, knowledge and kindness – surely the central ingredients of excellent dementia care for everyone.

We hope this book will give you the confidence to make sure that your own practice, and that of your colleagues, more than lives up to these expectations.

Prevalence

It is estimated that around 50 million people in the world live with a diagnosis of dementia, a number that is set to rise to 82 million in 2030 and 152 million in 2050 (World Health Organization, 2022). Because dementia does not discriminate, LGBTQ+ people are at least as likely as everyone else to develop dementia. Some of the stresses and strains associated with living as an LGBTQ+ person may increase the risk of dementia and may also increase the challenges of living with dementia (DiPlacido, 1998; Correro & Nielson, 2020).

How dementia affects LGBTQ+ people is not yet explored

or understood particularly well (McGovern, 2014; Westwood & Price, 2016; Baril & Silverman, 2019; Cousins, De Vries & Dening, 2021). There may be lots of reasons for this. Older LGBTQ+ people (dementia being an age-related condition) may not be 'out' (i.e. open about themselves) or may try to 'go back into the closet' (conceal themselves) if they need health and social care support. So, often dementia services do not know they have LGBTQ+ service users. Sometimes dementia services assume that their service users are heterosexual and/or cisgender, and simply do not ask the right questions to find out if people are LGBTQ+. This can also push LGBTQ+ people back 'into the closet' (Fish, 2006; Price, 2008; Almack, 2018; Löf & Olaison, 2020).

It is not clear how many LGBTQ+ people there are. The biggest reason for this is that not all of them are out and even those who are may not fill in forms or answer survey questions openly. Some are still fearful of how they will be perceived and how their information will be used. The UK government estimates that between 5 per cent and 7 per cent of people identify as lesbian, gay or bisexual (Stonewall, 2020a) although some suggest that it might be as much as 10 per cent of the population (Spiegelhalter, 2015). In terms of trans people, according to Stonewall (2020b), 'Government figures have tentatively suggested an estimate of 200,000 to 500,000 people but this figure isn't based on any robust data.'

LGBTQ+ people (who are a diverse population, with lots of differences among them) have different histories from non-LGBTQ+ people. They have lived their lives in different ways. Many have experienced oppression and social exclusion and the accumulative effects of this 'minority stress' have affected their health and wellbeing. Many have formed support networks with other LGBTQ+ people, as a way of compensating for exclusions from mainstream society. Many of them have 'families of friends' (Weston, 1997) which are as important, if not more important, than their families of origin. While some have children and grandchildren, fewer do than non-LGBTQ+ older people. Their cultures are often different and many have their own codes and signs and language that they share which are not common to non-LGBTQ+ people. The Pride annual celebrations of LGBTQ+ lives are important to many older LGBTQ+ people.

All these things, and more, need to be recognized, understood, respected and supported by dementia service providers. The aim of this book is to help people delivering care and support to LGBTQ+ people with dementia to achieve this.

> I stood at Pride last week. I was very moved, as I always am. I watched the armed forces go by and thought about all the women… who had been terribly oppressed in the armed forces, because they were suspected of being lesbians, or were sacked, or whatever. And I saw the teachers go by under their union banners, and I just wondered, and thought how impossible it would have been when I was a young teacher. And then I actually got very angry because, instead of thinking, oh how wonderful it is that it is different now, I thought, why did we have to put up with that crap? If it can be like this now, why did it ever have to be not like this? Because it damaged us. It limited our lives. *Audrey, lesbian, aged 67* (Westwood, 2016c, p.73)

How this chapter is structured
This chapter aims to give some background to the lives and contexts of LGBTQ+ people living with dementia, as follows:

- First, we briefly outline how the book is structured, and the different ways it can be used.

- Second, we offer a timeline of LGBTQ+ histories in the UK.

- Third, we explain the key concerns LGBTQ+ people have about dementia and dementia care.

- Lastly, we sum up the key learning points and offer some 'Food for thought' questions to encourage discussion and debate.

Book outline
The aim of this book is to identify what constitutes good practice in dementia care with LGBTQ+ people. We hope it will do more than simply enable individuals, teams, managers, services and organizations to identify and understand what good practice looks

like. We hope it will be used to reflect on practice, systems, policies and procedures which will, in turn, improve the care experiences of LGBTQ+ people living with dementia.

Each chapter has a similar structure, exploring a number of key issues enhanced by case examples and the voices of LGBTQ+ people themselves, some of whom are living with dementia. We include a 'Food for thought' section at the end of each chapter, with key questions to stimulate and encourage ongoing discussion and debate. We hope that this will also promote increased advocacy with and on behalf of LGBTQ+ people with dementia, their care partners and allies.

This chapter, **Chapter 1**, sets the scene, defining terms, giving a brief historical context, and outlining LGBTQ+ people's concerns.

Chapter 2 focuses on key areas of good practice in dementia care with LGBTQ+ people. It will be of particular interest to individuals and teams. We will emphasize the importance of inclusive language and an appreciation of diversity. We show how a 'sameness' approach to equality is not always enough.

Chapter 3 focuses on key policies, procedures and strategies necessary to facilitate and maintain LGBTQ-inclusive dementia care. It will be of particular interest to managers and leaders of organizations. We consider the importance of training and supervision and of ensuring that staff and teams feel safe and supported in dealing with LGBTQ+ issues. We highlight the importance of engaging with local LGBTQ+ organizations and including them in consultations and advisory groups and in the day-to-day service activities.

Chapter 4 considers some of the key challenges associated with advocating for, and supporting, LGBTQ+ people living with dementia and, most importantly, some strategies for how to overcome them. We consider how to engage with staff who disapprove of LGBTQ+ people in ways which may influence the quality of the care they provide. This includes addressing faith-based objections to LGBTQ+ people's rights; challenging commonplace misconceptions around issues of equality, most notably the idea that equality means 'treating everybody the same'; and challenging the belief that sexuality and gender identity should not be discussed because they are 'private matters'. It also involves considering ways to deal with other service users, their families and friends, if they have less than favourable attitudes towards LGBTQ+ people, especially in day, residential and home care contexts.

Chapter 5 sums everything up and offers pointers for next steps. This book offers some important information and ideas, but it is only the beginning for providers of dementia services and their journey towards LGBTQ+-inclusive dementia care.

There is a list of useful resources at the end of the book.

There was a sense from participants that cultural competence was as much a mindset as it was the possession of a set of skills, information and associated good practice. Being open minded, non-judgmental and assumption free were some of the ways in which care services could demonstrate and signal their inclusivity.

'Just being really willing to learn...some of my better care providers have just been open to being educated about it, it's not been about them having any prior knowledge but just being open to experiences and then going and educating themselves as a result.' *'Foxtrot', trans person* (Jones & Willis, 2016, p.9)

How to use this book
This book can be read in several ways. For those of you who want to get the overarching picture then the best way is to simply read it from beginning to end. Some of you may wish to start off with a chapter that is of particular interest to you, but in many ways, all of the book is relevant for everyone involved in the delivery of dementia care.

Key terms
LGBTQ+ – what's in an acronym?
You will, no doubt, be familiar with the LGBTQ+ acronym. You might, of course, identify with one or more of the groups under the LGBTQ+ umbrella yourself. If so, we hope the book offers you strategies for managing the challenges and sometimes difficult situations you will, no doubt, regularly face in your day-to-day work.

LGBTQ+ PEOPLE AND DEMENTIA

The LGBTQ+ acronym is certainly a very convenient, though sometimes awkward, way of referring collectively to lots of different minority sexuality and gender identity groups and individuals. It is a shorthand way of combining often very different groups of people (and individuals) who may have less in common than it first appears. The risk of using the shorthand is that we start assuming all LGBTQ+ people are the same and share the same issues and concerns, which they do not. For someone new to this area, it can feel a bit daunting coming to understand all the different terminology, especially as it is constantly changing. The simple solution is to ask someone how they identify.

> We want everyone to feel comfortable and supported as who they are when they need our care. It's vital that people are given the opportunity to be themselves from the first conversation. Healthcare professionals can make it easier for you to tell them – they can ask 'Who is important to you?' and 'What would you like to be called?'
> *Lauren, Marie Curie Nurse who identifies as LGBTQ+* (Marie Curie, 2020, p.6)

You will see in the Glossary at the end of the book, we have provided some of the key terms we will be using throughout the book, with their definitions.

Not all the same

As noted earlier, sometimes LGBTQ+ people are talked about as if they are all the same. But they're not! LGBTQ+ people have in common that they do not conform with gender and/or sexuality norms and stereotypes; however, they also differ in important ways. For example:

- Many lesbians and bisexual women are concerned about and affected by gender inequalities in ways which gay and bisexual men are not, particularly in relation to early socialization and experiences of sexism and sexual harassment (Westwood, 2016c).

- There can be exclusions among LGBTQ+ people. Some

older lesbians and gay men have little to do with one another because of the gendered differences among and between them (Westwood, 2017a). Many bisexual and trans people experience exclusions inside the 'LGBTQ+ community' as well as outside it (Jen & Jones, 2019).

- Many older gay and bisexual men have been affected by a long history of having to navigate criminalization, with an impact on their mental health, in ways which older lesbians and bisexual women did not experience (Hughes & Robinson, 2019).

- Many older LGBTQ+ people were affected by the AIDs crisis of the 1980s (Cant & Hemmings, 2010). Many lost friends and lovers during this time, and are still affected by this now. This disproportionately affected gay and bisexual men, some of whom are also ageing with HIV, which is now a chronic, as opposed to a fatal, condition (Rosenfeld, Bartlam & Smith, 2012). Current cohorts of older gay men are much smaller than they might have been because, sadly so many young gay and bisexual men died during the early years of the AIDs crisis.

- Many older gay men are excluded by ageism on the youth-privileging gay scene, in ways that other LGBTQ+ people do not experience (Simpson, 2013).

- While some trans people identify as lesbian, gay or bisexual and face the challenges of both minoritized sexualities and also trans-specific issues (Fredriksen-Goldsen *et al.*, 2014) others are straight (heterosexual) and only have limited shared concerns with lesbian, gay and bisexual people who are not trans (Sumerau *et al.*, 2018). Many older trans people have been deeply affected by lifelong transphobia and social exclusion specifically related to their gender identities.

Added to this, LGBTQ+ people come from all walks of life, all colours, races, ethnicities, cultures. Some are rich, some are poor, and many are somewhere in between, like most people. Some have big networks of family and friends. Some have smaller ones. Some are lonely and isolated. Some are not. Some have children and grandchildren. Some do not. Older lesbians are half as likely to have children compared with older heterosexual women, while heterosexual men are four times as likely to have children compared with gay men (Guasp, 2011).

(Older) LGBTQ+ people are a varied and diverse bunch of people, which is why a 'treating them all the same' approach to delivering services to them will not work.

One size doesn't fit all. *Martin, gay man, aged 62* **(Westwood, 2016c, p.135)**

LGBTQ+histories

The historical context within which older LGBTQ+ people, in particular, have lived their lives will give you an insight into the biographies which many LGBTQ+ people carry with them into, and beyond, the experience of living with dementia.

Older LGBTQ+ people in the UK have experienced significant changes in the law, as the following timeline shows.

There is no way we can give you a detailed history of LGBTQ+ lives in this book. To do so would take up the entire book. If you would like to know more, we suggest the following: Power (1995); Cant & Hemmings (2010). You can find these in the References section. However, it is important to make clear that older LGBTQ+ people now – those in their 60s, 70s, 80s, and 90s+ who are at greatest risk of age-related dementia – grew up and spent much of their adult lives during very different times. Those in their 90s were born in the 1930s, between the First World War and the Second World War. Some have memories of wartime Britain. Those in their 80s were born shortly before/during the Second World War. Those in their 60s and 70s were born into post-war Britain. During these times, there were still very strict codes for men's roles and women's roles, heterosexual marriage was very much the 'done thing' and LGBTQ+ lives were rarely talked about, or if they were it was disrespectfully.

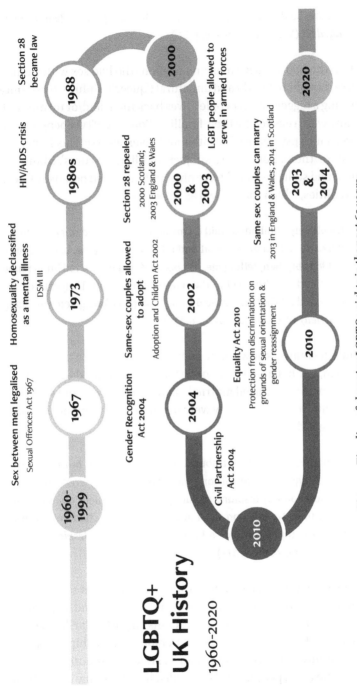

LGBTQ+
UK History
1960-2020

1960-1999

1967
Sex between men legalised
Sexual Offences Act 1967

1973
Homosexuality declassified as a mental illness
DSM III

1980s
HIV/AIDS crisis

1988
Section 28 became law

2000

2004
Civil Partnership Act 2004
Gender Recognition Act 2004

2002
Same-sex couples allowed to adopt
Adoption and Children Act 2002

2000 & 2003
Section 28 repealed
2000 Scotland; 2003 England & Wales

2003
LGBT people allowed to serve in armed forces

2010
Equality Act 2010
Protection from discrimination on grounds of sexual orientation & gender reassignment

2013 & 2014
Same sex couples can marry
2013 in England & Wales, 2014 in Scotland

2020

Figure 1: Timeline of changing LGBTQ+ rights in the past 60 years

> Mother said 'You're worse than a death in the family'. *Rene, lesbian, aged 63* (Westwood, 2016c, p.96)

Men who had sex with men and women who had sex with women were thought to be odd and unnatural ('queer'), sinful (Christianity playing a bigger role in people's lives back then) and/or mentally ill. Many were rejected by their families. Some LGBTQ+ people were forced into psychiatric hospitals and given electric shock therapy to 'cure' them. Some were subject to religious 'cures'. Many gay men (and some lesbians) were physically attacked because of their sexualities, which was known as 'queer bashing'.

> Oh blimey, I had hands laid on me and all sorts... I'd come out to my wife... to get rid of the devil and all that. Telling me, because we'd got kids by then, telling me...it's better if you have a rod hung round your neck, or drowned in the river or something. They quoted the Bible and all that. *Ian, aged 69, gay man (previously heterosexually married)* (Westwood, 2017b, p.374)

Some lesbians, knowing or suspecting they were attracted to women, got married (to men) because they wanted to have children. Some then stayed married. Some got divorced and some lost their children because they were deemed to be unfit mothers due to being lesbians.

> I always knew I was a lesbian... I knew how I felt. But my mother saw things on the television, and would then say 'Well, they were a whole load of lesbians anyway'. I thought, well, obviously it's going to be frowned on so... I got married, I had children, I wanted children anyway. It was a bit of a disaster. *Joan, lesbian, aged 67* (Westwood, 2016c, p.177)

Many lesbians and gay men built their own secret worlds – the 'gay scene' – where they could meet and socialize, and find romantic/sexual relationships. Many lesbians, in particular, lived below the radar, forming deep, hidden, personal friendships that have now endured across many decades (Traies, 2016, 2018).

Some trans people lived concealed lives for many years. Many suffered deep pain and associated poor mental health due to not being able to express their gender identities.

> [At 16–17 years] I thought, you know, I was a pervert, and this wasn't done... It was coming, well it came from the media. You were associated at that time with, um, homosexuality, you were associated with being a pervert, and that was the media as well as the people I mixed with at school. *Elaine, trans woman, aged 63* (Willis *et al.*, 2020, p.10)

Those who did come out as trans – in the many different ways that are possible – experienced social exclusion, attacks (some fatal), family rejection, and often lost their jobs.

> Most people that transition expect losses, sometimes a great many losses, but I didn't expect [to lose] everyone. I haven't heard from them since. For two years I desperately tried to connect with my family. And some of [the letters] weren't even opened. [The letters were returned saying] 'this person is dead' [images of letters with name struck out saying 'no such person!' and 'deceased']. It was horrible. It was vile. *KrysAnne, trans woman* (Riggs & Kentlyn, 2014, p.224)

Before 2000, although it was no longer a criminal offence for men to engage in consenting sexual activity, and although 'homosexuality' was no longer categorized as a mental illness, LGBTQ+ people still enjoyed fewer rights compared with the rest of the population.

> I was in the WRAF and I got kicked out. Well, I could've stayed in if I agreed to psychiatric treatment. But I said, there's nothing wrong with me, I'm not sick, I said, you can't change me, that's the way I am... I was 21. And I said, no, there's nothing wrong with me. I'm normal (laughs). So they said well you'll have to go then, so I said OK, I'll go. *Liz, gay, aged 52* (Westwood, 2016c, p.175)

Same-sex couples had no way for their relationships to be legally recognized. They were not allowed to adopt children. They were not allowed to serve in the armed forces, some losing their jobs if they were found out. Trans people were still classified as mentally ill (some still are, although now with a condition called gender dysphoria to which many trans people are deeply opposed (Sharpe, 2007)). They had no way of changing their legal gender.

'Section 28' – a time of repression and protest

In 1988, the Conservative government at the time, led by Margaret Thatcher, introduced 'Section 28' (under the Local Government Act 1988), which stated that local authorities 'shall not intentionally promote homosexuality or publish material with the intention of promoting homosexuality' nor 'promote the teaching in any maintained school of the acceptability of homosexuality as a pretended family relationship'. This had a devastating impact on LGBTQ+ people, with the government in effect silencing them and their voices, and denying them access to any information, guidance and support. Libraries removed any book that had anything connected to LGBTQ+ people or issues from their shelves. Teachers (many of whom were LGBTQ+ themselves) refused to discuss these issues with students (many of whom were also LGBTQ+) for fear of losing their jobs. The LGBTQ+ community, which had become increasingly politically active over several decades, campaigned vigorously to have Section 28 removed (Godfrey, 2018). It was eventually repealed in 2000 (Scotland) and 2003 (England and Wales). In 2009, a subsequent Conservative Prime Minister, David Cameron, apologized for the harm which had been caused by Section 28 (Watt, 2009).

> After Section 28 came in, there was certainly a difference in school environments. A lot of teachers did not want to deal with the subject out of fear. Bigoted teachers were emboldened. A lot of schools pretended that homosexuality did not exist and it allowed a lot of misinformation, prejudice and abuse to go unchallenged. And, of course, it had a terrible effect on young people: students suffered homophobic abuse in silence and teachers and schools did nothing about it. *Michael Dance, gay, a teacher at the time of Section 28* (Godfrey, 2018)

The new millennium – a new era of progress?

Since 2000, there have been dramatic legal changes affecting LGBTQ+ people. They can now openly serve in the armed forces. Same-sex couples can now adopt. Same-sex couples can now form civil partnerships and get married, though if they want a religious service they will need to find a religious organizations which has 'opted in' to doing so, and not all have. For older LGBTQ+ people this was particularly important, both for the validation and social respectability it gave them. It was also because they could legally be involved in one another's care, and in end-of-life decision-making, and take control of their partner's funeral when they died, very often having previously being excluded.

> I knew he wanted a burial and he wanted to be buried next to his mother. He ended up being cremated [which] was totally against his religion... I couldn't stop them but it was like strangers organizing his funeral; I was his family... But he never wanted it to be known that he was gay. (Marie Curie, 2017, p.29)

Under the Gender Recognition Act 2004, people can now change their legal gender, although many trans people think it too bureaucratic and that it does not go far enough (Fairbairn, Pyper & Balogun, 2022), and laws may change in the various devolved nations in this regard.

A new legal framework

The Equality Act 2010 protects nine 'characteristics' from direct and indirect discrimination, harassment and victimization. Two of the protected characteristics are 'sexual orientation' and 'gender reassignment' (subsequently established in a 2020 legal case[2] to include gender fluid and gender non-binary people). The Act covers a wide range of contexts, including health and social care provision. Under the Act's Public Sector Equality Duty, public bodies are required to: eliminate unlawful discrimination,

---

2   Ms R Taylor v Jaguar Land Rover Ltd: 1304471/2018: www.gov.uk/employment-tribunal-decisions/ms-r-taylor-v-jaguar-land-rover-ltd-1304471-2018

harassment and victimization and other conduct prohibited by the Act; advance equality of opportunity and foster good relations between people who share a protected characteristic and those who do not; remove or minimize disadvantages suffered by people due to their protected characteristics; take steps to meet the specific needs of people from protected groups; encourage people from protected groups to participate in public life. This now places a legal expectation on services to become more inclusive of minority groups, including LGBTQ+ people.

It is clear from this very brief overview that the social, legal and political attitudes towards LGBTQ+ people have shifted significantly in recent decades. The fact remains, however, that, for older people in particular, life stories founded on exclusion, marginalization and oppression will have a lasting legacy. LGBTQ+ people have been variously labelled mentally sick, weak, perverted, sinners, criminals, a public menace and, at best, the unfortunate victims of delayed development. So, for LGBTQ+ people who are now ageing, the legacy of this historical narrative is one which endures, leaving lasting feelings of shame and the perceived need to conceal their identity, despite some of the social and political changes which have meant, at least, a rhetorical softening of attitudes. It is, then, this ongoing narrative which, inevitably, goes on to shape the experience of dementia.

It is clear, also, that there is a growing cohort of younger people who have lived in far more liberal times and for whom the negative legacy of the past is far less pressing. For them, the experience of ageing and, for some, the experience of dementia, will, of course, be different. Their experience of dementia will, as we will argue throughout the book, continue to be very much shaped by public and political attitudes which can be less than accommodating to anyone who does not conform to heterosexual and/or gender norms. Indeed, this younger cohort of people will reasonably demand dementia care which both acknowledges and validates their sexualities and gender identities. Thus, for both older and younger LGBTQ+ people alike, there is a pressing need for dementia care service providers to be able to respond appropriately, and sensitively, to LGBTQ+ people.

I live in an incredible amount of fear about my future. Not just as an older person. But as a gay older person. Institutions, they're very straight. My god I hope I don't have to go into a care home, I really do... When I think about it, I find it quite scary. It frightens me that I am just going to be invisible, a nobody, that I am just going to be lost. And what I would want to do is just die. *May, gay woman, aged 64* (Westwood, 2016c, p.138)

LGBTQ+ people and dementia care – key issues

This book will help you to understand and address some of the issues which impact on LGBTQ+ people living with dementia. As we have noted above, LGBTQ+ people's biographies are shaped differently from those of the majority population and these biographies endure into old age and beyond. It is important to recognize, then, that older LGBTQ+ people are less likely than their heterosexual or cisgender counterparts to enjoy supportive relationships with their biological family. In this context, for some older LGBTQ+ people, the 'family of choice' (the group of people who fulfil a person's 'family' needs but who are not biologically related) may well constitute much of their support network. With the onset of some of the conditions of older age, such as dementia, however, this model can generate its own difficulties:

> While 'families of choice' do provide social support, a key problem that older LGB people may face is that members of their 'family of choice' may be the same age as them and so this network of family/friends is likely to have age related problems at the same time and may not be as effective at providing the social support that may be necessary. (Musingarimi, 2008, p.4)

When it comes to needing formal support, LGBTQ+ people with dementia, and their friends and family, may be fearful about the response to their sexuality and/or gender identity from care providers, and, given the discrimination and stigma many LGBTQ+ people have faced in their lifetimes, they may be very reticent about accessing and receiving support in the context of their dementia. In particular, the onset of dementia may create additional difficulties when maintaining hard-won personal privacy. Previous private living arrangements and relationships might suddenly be forced into the public domain and opened up to public scrutiny.

> In the residential home in which the person she [lesbian interviewee] and her partner cared for was resident... she was effectively 'outed' when they went to visit the person they cared for who would say [quoting interviewee]: 'Oh, that's right, how long have you two been together?' And I'm like oh, God, shut up, you know... And I could see out of the corner of my eye the whole staff turns round! (Price, 2010, p.166)

For trans people in particular, requiring personal care from others can generate very particular anxieties and concerns (Witten, 2016; Hunter, Bishop & Westwood, 2016; Baril & Silverman, 2019).

> I worry that I will become incapacitated and not be able to com-municate my history as a trans person (medical, surgical history) before requiring care. I worry that caregivers will not be experi-enced in dealing with trans bodies and health issues and I will at best not get the care I need and at worst be ridiculed, mocked and ignored because of the state of my body. *Transgender MetLife Survey respondent* (Witten, 2016b, p.203)

In this context, trans people's fears and anxieties revolve around both their physical and gender presentation. Indeed, research in this area is replete with distressing stories which highlight, starkly, the very real fears that trans people have in relation to receiving care. The realities of living with dementia only serve, of course, to heighten and underpin these anxieties.

For lesbian, gay and bisexual people, too, there are significant anxieties associated with requiring care, particularly in supported living contexts where fears are associated with heteronormative environments in nursing/care homes (where heterosexuality is the norm and other sexualities are, at best, tolerated or oth-erwise ignored). At worst, of course, there can be open hostil-ity to LGBTQ+ people from both the residents and care staff, particularly, research suggests, from those who ascribe to certain deeply held religious beliefs.

> There is a severe lack of understanding about the particular needs of older lesbian and gay people, especially from some faith-based organizations that provide care services. *John, 57, London, UK* (Guasp, 2011, p.11)

Unsurprisingly, therefore, research suggests that when care is required, older LGBTQ+ people would prefer to be cared for in their own homes, but failing that, they would like an environment which is 'LGBTQ+ friendly'. Many older lesbians, particularly those who have lived their lives in women-only communities, would like to be cared for in women-only/lesbian-only environments (Westwood, 2017a).

> Everything is predominantly heterosexual orientated. Sheltered and residential housing is mixed with no provision for those who prefer the company of their own orientation. It's depressing to think I might end up in a home where I could be isolated because to disclose/talk about my life would lead to ostracization. *Molly, 68* (Guasp, 2011, p.27)

The following is the first of several case examples we will be providing in this book, which demonstrate good practice in delivering dementia care to LGBTQ+ people.

GOOD PRACTICE EXAMPLE 1.1

What does LGBTQ+-inclusive dementia care look like?

Sue [pseudonym] had been living at her care home in rural Durham for a while when staff noticed how confused and agitated she was becoming about her gender identity. Diagnosed with a variant of Alzheimer's just before her 60th birthday, Sue...had to move into residential care when her symptoms progressed...staff grew more worried as Sue began to refer to herself as 'Cliff'... She would become distressed by her appearance and unsettled by her physicality. These episodes became more frequent and the care home was at a loss as to how to support her.

Because care managers had no contact with Sue's family and no idea of her medical history, they were unaware that she was a trans woman. Sue had been estranged from her family since they had rejected her following her decision to transition in the late 1970s. She had completed gender reassignment surgery at the age of 42. A social worker at the care home sought the support and advice of [a local LGBT organization] on how to work with Sue and remain sensitive to her gender identity.

[The organization] formed a partnership group between the local authority social services and Sue's GP – who was the only one who knew her medical history. [They worked together] to collaborate on a new care plan. Using memory books and encouraging a personal sense of gender, the plan reinforced Sue's identity.

In addition, care home staff received awareness training on trans identities, including the impact of stigma and misgendering – being labelled by someone as having a gender other than the one you identify with...

As Sue's dementia became more severe, staff were able to offer her appropriate care and support, confident in the knowledge that their approach was tailored to her very personal needs and gender history. Not only did this approach benefit Sue's wellbeing and quality of life, but all the partners involved in her care plan gained a stronger understanding of the issues faced by trans service users and delivered more empathic care.

Through their experience with Sue, health, care and social services staff developed their knowledge and skills around LGBT people's needs, and are using this to improve their and care provision for other people they support in the future.

National Care Forum (2016, pp.7–8)

This case study highlights a number of important strategies used to support a trans woman with dementia, many of which can be applied in relation to all LGBTQ+ people. It demonstrates the importance of understanding the perspective of a person with dementia, and of locating that perspective in context. It also highlights how helpful it can be to work with local community organizations, which can, in turn, facilitate more joined-up working.

Most of all it emphasizes that care teams do not have to be experts on LGBTQ+ ageing, they just have to reach out to get the specialist guidance and support they need. At the heart of this example of good practice is something very simple: the care team recognized that they did not understand enough about the person they were trying to help, and so they went and found some people to help them understand. By doing so, they also became more skilled and knowledgeable, which informed their future practice.

Conclusion

As this chapter has shown, it is important, as practitioners and as service providers, to understand the specific, and diverse, needs of LGBTQ+ people with dementia because they may differ significantly from those of the majority heterosexual population. Good practice in dementia care involves person-centred care, which emphasizes seeing the person with dementia as an individual in their unique context (Manthorpe & Samsi, 2016). Getting dementia services 'right' for minority populations means that they will be right for everyone (Ward, Pugh & Price, 2010). We are currently quite a long way away from a place where all dementia service provision is LGBTQ+inclusive. However, as the case study shows, there is good practice out there. We hope this book will arm you with ideas and strategies to help you to develop your own inclusive practice with LGBTQ+ people with dementia and to enable you to challenge discriminatory values, views and practice when you come across them.

FOOD FOR THOUGHT

- Why are sexuality and gender identity important – what difference do they make to living with dementia?
- Do you think your organization is willing to learn about

how to recognize, understand, respect and support the various needs of LGBTQ+ people with dementia?

- Do you think there might be any reluctance in your organization to tackle these issues? If so, does this need to be addressed? How?

- What do you personally need to do to learn about the needs of LGBTQ+ people with dementia (in addition to reading this book)?

KEY LEARNING POINTS

✓ Fifty million people currently live with dementia, and this is predicted to rise to 82 million in 2030 and 152 million in 2050.

✓ LGBTQ+ people are affected by dementia in ways which are sometimes the same as non-LGBTQ+ people, and sometimes different.

✓ Not all LGBTQ+ people are the same.

✓ Older LGBTQ+ people have complex and often traumatic histories which make them very wary of health and social care services, especially dementia care.

✓ LGBTQ+ people need dementia services that recognize, understand, respect and support the different aspects of their needs.

Chapter 2

Good Practice in Dementia Care with LGBTQ+ People

Chapter summary

This chapter:

- ✓ explains how to *recognize, understand, respect and support LGBTQ+ people with dementia*

- ✓ invites you to think carefully about *why 'equality' does not always mean treating everyone the same way*

- ✓ discusses what *LGBTQ+-affirmative care* looks like

- ✓ suggests *ways to create welcoming environments for LGBTQ+ people* with dementia

- ✓ may be of particular interest to individuals and teams delivering services to people with dementia.

Introduction

This chapter explores what it means to recognize, understand and support LGBTQ+ people with dementia, highlighting their main concerns. We offer case examples of good practice. As they show, this does not have to involve big things. Often small gestures mean a lot, and it is the thinking behind the actions that is as important, if not more important, than the actions themselves. Later in the chapter we think about LGBTQ+-affirmative care and what this means. But first we explore how treating everyone equally does not mean always treating them same way.

Sometimes you have to treat people differently, to treat them equally

> I've got dementia so I shouldn't be ashamed of being gay and coming out and talking to somebody about it. And who's there to talk to, you know, the danger is that you set people up... lot of people would say...but we deal with everyone in a person-centred way and we treat everybody as if they're equal. And that is good that we treat everybody the same but what I'm hearing...is actually we don't want to be treated the same because you're saying the same is assuming that we're heterosexual. And that's really...so actually I do want to be treated differently. *June* (Peel & McDaid, 2015, p.14)

So, you're on a training day. It is the afternoon. You have had lunch, which was very nice. But no drinks were provided, which you thought was a bit odd. Now you are thirsty. The organizers say drinks will be served in the training room. Good, you think. Back in the training room, everyone is ready for those drinks. The organizers bring in trays, and start handing out mugs to everyone. A mug comes your way. It is hot. You sniff it. Coffee with milk. Ugh, you hate coffee. You call out, 'Excuse me, I don't drink coffee.' Someone else calls out, 'I don't take milk.' Another person says, 'Is there any sugar?' Someone says, 'I don't drink hot drinks.' 'Ah,' says the organizer with a smile, 'But I am just treating you all equally. I am just treating you all the same.'

This is the problem with taking a 'sameness' approach to equality. We are not all the same, and we need our different needs and wishes respected and validated. We should all be treated *equally well*, and sometimes that means being treated in different ways.

Treating a lesbian, gay or bisexual person as if they are heterosexual, or a trans person as if they are cisgender, ignores their identities, the lives they have lived, their histories and, for some of them, their sub-cultures. To treat them equally as well as their heterosexual and/or cisgender counterparts, you need to appreciate that they are not all the same. The important thing is to understand how individuals see themselves, to try to see things from their point of view, and to get to know what and who is important to them. Then you can begin to appreciate what they need from you to deliver them an equally good service.

Similarly, not all lesbians, gay men, bisexual women or men are all the same. There are a lot of differences between older lesbians in particular (Traies, 2016, 2018; Westwood, 2016c). Some 'always knew' they were lesbian/gay. Some denied it, even to themselves. Some knew but married men so they could have children. For some lesbians, it gradually dawned on them across their adult lives, and some only discovered it very late in life. Some lesbians 'gave up' men in the 1970s and 1980s, as part of their feminist politics.

> My trans colleague Jenny-Anne and I (both lesbians) see the world in very different ways. She loves it when she is called 'Madam' and when men hold the door open for her, whereas I say to her I have spent my whole life trying to stop them! *Sue, 64, lesbian (co-author) (identifies with her birth sex)*

For many older lesbians, their communities of friendship with women and other older lesbians are essential for their wellbeing (Traies, 2015). Some have children and grandchildren, but some do not, and for many lesbians, this can be an important difference.

> There is an expectation (in the media and in government planning, I think) that everyone has family even if they don't live with you. But I don't – no children, siblings, parents, grandparents etc. *Lesbian/ gay woman, age bracket 70–74* (Westwood, Hafford-Letchfield & Toze, 2021a, p.24)

By contrast, most gay men say they have always known they were gay, even though it took some a long time to admit it even to themselves. Some older gay men are still active on the gay scene, where there can be a lot of ageism, while others are not (Simpson, 2013). Some have built networks away from the scene, but some have not, and they can experience profound loneliness and social isolation in later life (Guasp, 2011).

Many lesbians and gay men have been with their long-term partners (often now civil partners or wives/husbands) for decades. Some have lived highly concealed lives. When a partner dies, it can, of course, leave the surviving partner bereft (Bristowe, Marshall & Harding, 2016), particularly if they have some sort of memory loss, which often gets worse following bereavement.

> Other gay men respondents also differentiated between older gay men in couples, single older men who have 'retired' from the gay commercial scene and those who are still involved in it: 'It's more a generational split. Or between people who are still in market for sex and those who gave it up years ago.' *Gay man, age bracket 65–69* (Westwood, Hafford-Letchfield & Toze, 2021b, p.38)

Bisexual people are not all the same, and they are affected differently by both ageing and by dementia (Witten, 2016b; Jones, Almack & Scicluna, 2016, 2018; Jen & Jones, 2019). One of the unique challenges they face is in telling histories which involve partners of both genders, as this can result in biphobic prejudice and discrimination.

Similarly, trans people (many of whom are also bisexual, Jen & Jones, 2019) are very diverse and have a whole host of different needs (Hunter, Bishop & Westwood, 2016). For those who have not transitioned, their bodies may not align with their gender identities, which can raise particular issues for personal care (Witten, 2016b). Others may not identify with gender at all. Care staff need to be open to some individuals living with gender in different ways from the majority population. Most of all, trans people want to be accepted for who they are (Willis *et al.*, 2020).

> It's a whole spectrum and you can't just get locked into one story and be like 'OK, I know, you grew up in the wrong body and now you're in the right gender and you're finally happy, I get it' because it's not that way for everybody. *'Golf', a trans person* (Jones & Willis, 2016, p.7)

Recognition, understanding, respect and support
Recognition

> Jane lives in a care home in the Calder Valley and has dementia. There was no discussion of sexuality at the admission stage. Jane kept asking for people. They were all women's names, Jane called one name repeatedly. When asked by staff, Jane's next of kin, a much younger brother, explained it this way: 'When I was growing up I had a lot of aunties.' The oft repeated name is Jane's partner. 'She has her own problems and lives in another care home nearby.' Two separate families decided that they should live in two separate care homes. *Care Home Manager Interview* (Walker *et al.*, 2013, p.25)

Sometimes, when staff attend training on delivering services to LGBTQ+ people with dementia, one of the first things they say is, 'We don't have any here'. And we will respond, 'How do you know?' Many services do not ask people how they identify in terms of their sexual orientation or gender identity. Some people and organizations think it is a 'private matter'.

> I think there needs to be more of a realization that people are gay because there is an assumption that everyone is straight. You know, I'm forever being called Mrs somebody or other. Just to think about it before they assume. And my partner would not be amused by me saying this but she's older than me, so we've got nearly 19 years of an age gap; I think a lot of people do assume she's my mother, actually. *Lynda, lesbian, 64* (Marie Curie, 2017, p.25)

If you don't have a mechanism to ask if someone is LGBTQ+, you will not give them the opportunity to tell you, and, importantly, you give the impression that you do not understand that this is important (Westwood, 2017b; Marie Curie, 2017).

> [Clifford's partner had just died, and he asked for a priest, because that is what he thought his partner would have wanted. The priest arrived and...] When we were doing the pleasantries, he kept saying,

'Shall we go and see your friend', as though it was just that, and I thought we can't go on like this, sort of beating about the bush, really, so I said, 'He is my friend, my best friend, my lover, we've been together for 33 years.' … I mean, he'd just died, and I wasn't going to let anybody devalue our relationship… And there was a bit of shuffling and sort of taking stock. But after that he was actually quite good. *Clifford, aged 68* (Westwood, 2017b, p.64)

Recognizing that someone *might* identify as LGBTQ+ does not involve trying to 'spot' someone who is. It is about being open to the possibility that someone *could* be. This means you should use language and ask questions in ways which do not make presumptions about a person's sexuality or gender identity.

GOOD PRACTICE EXAMPLE 2.1

I always talk in terms of 'those who are important to you' as opposed to 'family' so I am open to that being whoever it is. The key for me is asking the patient.

(Marie Curie, 2017, p.34)

Even if services do ask, many LGBTQ+ people, especially older people, may not answer honestly because they do not know if it is safe to do so.

GOOD PRACTICE EXAMPLE 2.2

It is not always possible to know someone's gender based on their name or how they look or sound. This is the case for all people, not just transgender people. When addressing patients we don't know, we can accidentally call them by the wrong gender, causing embarrassment. One way to prevent this mistake is by addressing people without using any terms that indicate a gender. For example, instead of asking 'How may I help you, sir?' you can simply ask, 'How may I help you?' You can also avoid using 'Mr./Mrs./Miss/Ms.' by calling someone by their first name (if this is an acceptable practice in your organization) or by using their first and last name together. You can also avoid using a person's name by tapping the person on the shoulder and saying, for example, 'Excuse me, we're ready for you now. Please come this way.'

(National LGBT Center 2013, p.6)

LGBTQ+ people often do not easily fit into boxes (as all individuals do not) so it is important to think outside the box when ensuring that services are open and ready to meet their needs.

> As someone who identified as a cross-dresser, Dolly expressed con-
> cerns about living with dementia and the difficulty of conveying
> a non-transitioning status to care workers: 'If someone goes into
> a home, at some point in the future, and they start to suffer from
> dementia ... there wouldn't necessarily be anything in place for me,
> because I don't identify in a medical way, therefore, if I suddenly
> started expressing a preference to do certain things or to present
> myself in a certain way, are the care workers going to say, "It's just
> part of the dementia"?'
> Dolly described being 'a non-transitioning person' as a grey area
> where care workers and services are unsure how to categorize and
> respond to one's needs and wellbeing: 'If you take yourself out of
> one bucket, you put yourself in the other one, they know how to
> deal with you. Society's not very good at dealing with grey areas.'
> Dolly, 54 (Willis *et al.*, 2020, p.15)

Part of being open to people possibly identifying under the LGBTQ+ umbrella is not making assumptions.

> They don't ask you about your sexuality, they ask about your het-
> erosexuality: 'Do you have children?'...which is not an offence. It's a
> simple question. But it creates that tiny little bit of distance...which
> is saying, 'I'm heterosexual and I wonder what your experience of
> heterosexuality is...' And it's perfectly fair, it doesn't offend me or
> anything like that. But it says I'm different. Basically it's...speaking
> in ways that assume that you already share that sexuality, rather
> than coming at the topic with an open mind that you might be gay.
> Andrew, 67, gay man (Walker *et al.*, 2013, p.25)

One of the ways you can show you recognize LGBTQ+ people is to make sure they can see themselves in your care environment. This means having posters and pictures of LGBTQ+ people and same-sex couples on the walls; videos and DVDs which are about LGBTQ+ people; LGBTQ+ 'classics' in your book collection; leaflets and information booklets with LGBTQ+-specific information, including about local LGBTQ+ social events and support groups; posters of Pride, and information about local Pride events, displayed; rainbow flags displayed; and signs which make it clear that 'This is an LGBTQ+-friendly environment' and 'We provide LGBTQ+-inclusive care'.

> ...in care homes I think as well. There's got to be some signs around, that you know, people can pick up on, there could be pictures on the wall of same-sex people or whatever. I mean I would do very much more than that but I'm just thinking of what an up-hill battle it is with care homes. *Arnold* (Peel & McDaid, 2015, p.19)

It is important to ensure that LGBTQ+ people have access to cultural resources (books, videos, magazines, music) which resonate with their personal/cultural histories.

> I don't want to be sitting in [an] older person's home with a lot of straight people singing Second World War songs. I'd rather be sitting with people that I can relate to, watching gay cabaret, or getting some of the LGBT film festival films coming in, you know, that sort of thing. *Alice, aged 60, lesbian* (Westwood, 2016c, p.139)

This can go a long way to allaying LGBTQ+ people's fears (as long as it is also backed up by good practice). This sends a clear message to everyone – staff, service users, their family, friends and other visitors – that the service is truly committed to LGBTQ+-inclusive care.

GOOD PRACTICE EXAMPLE 2.3

'Safety signals'
Safety signals are...messages that other people send...regarding the safety of disclosure... For some, this involved appraising others'

attitudes to determine if they were receptive. Eleanor and Jack suggested that their doctor stopping to visit indicated receptiveness. Eleanor explained: 'They said what relationship are you and I said we're partners and he said that's fine. He's so nice to me. When he drives past he stops to talk to me and everything.'

Yvonne [said] '…If I'm not sure, you know, what the attitude of the other person is. I would wait until I get to know them and trust them.'

For Laurie and Rose, verbal acceptance of their sexual orientation from others indicated safety, while for Frank these signals could be non-verbal. He and Louis attended a carers group and continued receiving a warm welcome after revealing their relationship.

(McParland & Camic, 2018, p.466)

Understanding

LGBTQ+ people with dementia need and deserve to be cared for and supported by people who understand them. You need to get to know each person as an individual, of course. But knowing a little about LGBTQ+ histories (see Chapter 1) and key terms (see the Glossary) is a good start.

What also needs to be understood are issues relating to appearance. Some lesbians are 'femme' (feminine in appearance) and some are 'butch' (masculine in appearance). To put a 'femme' woman in 'butch' clothing will cause her distress. Likewise, to put a butch woman in feminine clothes (e.g. a dress, rather than trousers) will cause her distress.

One woman gives an example of a lesbian friend with dementia she knew who had always worn trousers being put in a crimplene dress and given a standard 'old woman's perm'. (Knocker, 2012, p.12)

For trans people, there are many different ways that they need care providers to be both prepared for, and supportive of, their diversity. Trans people who need personal care may be very worried that staff will be shocked and embarrassed, and, worse, might even laugh at and humiliate them.

I am a woman with a penis. What will they do to me in a nursing home? What will happen if I cannot defend myself because of dementia? *Anonymous Transgender MetLife Survey respondent* (Witten, 2016b, p.136)

One of the things you have to do with a vaginoplasty[1] is that you have to dilate the vagina with a medical stent on a regular basis, every two weeks indefinitely for the rest of your life...what if I get to the point where I'm physically not as able to do that for myself? How do I talk to them about that? I mean it's obviously going to be an awkward conversation. *'Echo', trans person* (Jones & Willis, 2016, p.9)

For trans women and men who have transitioned, to be dressed in clothing for their old legal gender is not only traumatic, but misgenders them and is contrary to the Equality Act 2010.

GOOD PRACTICE EXAMPLE 2.4

Sometimes small choices can make a big difference. For example, if a trans man in a nursing home has feet that are too small for men's slippers, rather than buying women's slippers, service providers should purchase boy's slippers instead.

(AGE UK, 2011, p.24)

LGBTQ+ people with memory loss need to reminisce, like all people with memory loss do, but they cannot do that reminiscing with people who do not have a basic understanding of what they are talking about and respect for who they are.

It's about people, you know, gay and lesbian people being able to talk about their lives, and feel people are interested and that. Cos it's really important to reminisce, you know. *Jack, aged 66, gay man* (Westwood, 2016c, p.146)

To put an LGBTQ+ person in a group of exclusively non-LGBTQ+

---

1   A vaginoplasty is a procedure to construct or repair a vagina.

people not only exposes them to the risk of homophobia, but also means that they will not have anyone else in the group they can identify with. This could make them feel even more lonely, isolated and confused.

> Being in care or being in an old people's home and being the only gay woman – that is quite a daunting prospect, that is – because one of the things that is important really isn't it – is remembering things and talk, isn't it? *Gail, older lesbian* (Pugh, 2012, p.45)

Trans people also need particularly sensitive support when staff are doing reminiscence work with them. Some trans women and men who have transitioned are very worried that they may not remember they have done so. Creating memory books reminding them about their transitioning can help in this regard.

> I am worried that I will develop dementia and will not remember that I have transitioned. *Anonymous Transgender MetLife Survey respondent* (Witten, 2016b, p.136)

Language is crucial when supporting a trans person, and it needs to be used very carefully when doing memory work. A trans woman will have grown up as a little boy; a trans man as a girl. It is important to get the pronoun's right and not 'misgender' someone, i.e. call them 'he' when it should be 'she' or vice versa. And this mistake can be made very easily, when you are talking about 'he' the little boy, and 'she' the adult, for example.

> How do you do that positively? If you're doing sort of reminiscence or asking people to talk about when they were younger and they may have had much clearer memories. How you do that in a positive, supportive way? [referring to talking about a trans woman's childhood] Do you talk about, I mean if [you] don't know [that she is transgender] then you would say 'when you were a little girl', but [she was] a little boy. How you do that in a positive way, that's kind of reinforcing and recognizing the journey and the transition, but that's not confusing to them and not confusing to the staff. I mean, it's really quite a delicate thing that needs to be thought out really

carefully, doesn't it?' *Bethan* (Peel & McDaid, 2015, p.12) (Talking about memory work with a trans woman.)

Some trans women and trans men transition in early adulthood. Others, especially trans women (Bouman *et al.*, 2016), may not transition until very late in life, having spent much of their lives living as (although not feeling like) a man. Some are rejected by their families as a consequence. Not all trans people identify with the gender binary (i.e. as female or male). There needs to be support and understanding for these issues, because reminiscence for them is often complicated and full of risks of inadvertently causing distress.

Looking back on the past, for many LGBTQ+ people, means looking back on trauma, stigma, rejection and persecution, and the risk is that memory work can re-traumatize them (Cousins, De Vries & Dening, 2021). So, it needs to be done in a very carefully thought-through way (Concannon, 2009; Pugh, 2012; Carr & Ross, 2013).

Respect

All care regulators require that care providers must treat people with dignity and respect. Respecting LGBTQ+ people means more than being polite and courteous, or even kind and compassionate. Respecting an LGBTQ+ person involves truly valuing their humanity and regarding them as having equal worth to everyone else. It means supporting and validating their lives, relationships and identities.

Ann was living at home and had a worker assisting her to shower because her partner Mary was no longer able to help her. Last week the worker asked if they were lesbians. Mary denied that they were because she was concerned that Ann would receive a lesser standard of care. However, one morning the care worker noticed they had both been sleeping in the double bed. The care worker refused to touch Ann in the shower. Mary was concerned because Ann needed a lot of assistance and she couldn't understand why the care worker wouldn't help. Ann was confused and distressed and Mary thought about ringing the service provider to make a report, but she didn't know what she should say. (Birch, 2009, p.22)

Sometimes LGBTQ+ people experience prejudice and discrimination, and this can have a detrimental effect on their wellbeing.

> An older gay man with dementia decided to stop receiving services because of the homophobic reaction of care staff. This had led to him having to move into residential care earlier than necessary as his elderly partner had struggled to cope alone with caring responsibilities. (Equality & Human Rights Commission, 2011, p.37)

Sometimes, LGBTQ+ people feel that staff talk about them in disrespectful ways.

> Muriel is 78. [She has had relationships in the past with both women and men] Last year, Joan [her partner] died and Muriel...started receiving home care. She gets on well with one of her regular carers who asks her about the photos she has up around the house of her former partners [both women and men]. Muriel answers honestly but is horrified to discover later that her carer has spread malicious gossip among her colleagues about her past, saying that Muriel had been sexually predatory and promiscuous. (Hypothetical scenario described by Jones, 2016, p.4)

Sometimes, trans people feel their trans-specific issues are not dealt with sufficient discretion and concern for their privacy.

> I've been in [hospital]...where it has 10 bays with 10 patients, just with curtains. And you can hear every conversation... Some doctors have said to me, 'How long have you been transgendered for?' and everybody has heard. *Louise, 51, trans woman* (Marie Curie, 2017, p.25)

GOOD PRACTICE EXAMPLE 2.5

For transgender individuals, respect must be shown for their identity and history, for their personal style (clothes, accessories, etc.), for their bodily configuration, and for their name and pronoun. Respect extends beyond direct interactions to include what you say and how you behave *even outside of their presence.*

(FORGE, 2011, p.1)

Sometimes LGBTQ+ people have reported that some health and social care staff who are extremely religious have said or done things which are not respectful.

> I've heard a care worker say 'Oh pray for them', if they're gay or refuse to touch their body. Because they might, if it's gay men then they'll get AIDS, um, if it's gay women it might be taken wrong or want you to interfere with them, um, you know as if we've got not taste at all...but a lot of them actually hide their sexuality when the carer's there. They literally change the room where the carer's going to come into, taking photographs, the whole room, and put it all back out again afterwards. *Josie* (Peel & McDaid, 2015, p.13)

> One older disabled lesbian woman describes being given leaflets by religious care workers suggesting that she could be 'saved'; an experience that has made her feel unsafe and alienated in her own home. (Knocker, 2012, p.10)

Sometimes LGBTQ+ staff also experience discrimination.

> I was told I should be hanging from a tree by a nurse from Nigeria with strong religious beliefs. People refused to drink from a mug I had used in case I had AIDS. *Chris, Nurse, North West* (Stonewall, 2015, p.6)

This is not always the case, of course. Many staff, including religious staff, are LGBTQ+ people themselves (Westwood, 2017b) and many religious staff who are not LGBTQ+ nonetheless deliver very good care.

GOOD PRACTICE EXAMPLE 2.6

It was one of the hospice chaplains that still brings back some warmth to the memory; she walked into the room, introduced herself and just sat with Diane. She did not want to know if she had any affiliations religiously, and then for some reason just said, 'I can sing something if you would like'. Diane nodded. This lady then sang Diane's favourite piece of religious music, John Rutter's 'The Lord

Bless You and Keep You'. It was already in her memory book for her thanksgiving service. She held her hand and just sang... The upshot was she saw the person, which included recognizing our relationship. Holistic care is about the whole person; it does not have to be a man or woman with a collar on, it can be anyone who can understand that we are at our closest to faith and/or our own spirituality when facing death. It's made so much harder by the failure of those who provide care to recognize our humanity, regardless of the gender of the person we have dedicated our lives to. *Carol, 57, partner of Diane*

(Marie Curie, 2017, p.23)

Support
Support for LGBTQ+ people with dementia means more than just supporting their dementia-related needs. It means supporting them holistically, for all of who they are.

> You don't stop being lesbian or gay if you're not in a sexual relation-ship... I mean for me, my identity is lesbian whatever I'm doing. If I'm choosing what to watch on the tellie, choosing what to wear on holiday, it's not all about, you know, sex. There's so much else and that's the message I would like to get across. Actually, by the time you go into a nursing home or something, actually the last thing you're thinking about is having sex. And the carers shouldn't be thinking about what if they have sex, it's just about preserving this person's identity and remembering who they are and remembering their whole life's history as somebody with an identity which is lesbian and gay. *Bethan* (Peel & McDaid, 2015, p.8)

Central to LGBTQ+-affirmative care is good care planning which should identify and plan for the things a person likes to do, the people who are important to them, and how contact with them will be maintained.

> If I'm in a sheltered unit or an old people's home, I want to be able to read and get information and I want to be able to connect with my community. I want to go to [older lesbian group] still. Now how am I going to get to [older lesbian group] if my mobility is

compromised? Is somebody going to get me a special bus? If I'm lucky I'll have friends who'll take me there once a month. But what if I have Alzheimer's? Will it be assumed I'm heterosexual and I don't need my friends to come and talk to me about my past? *Diana, aged 69, lesbian* (Westwood, 2015b, p.1506)

GOOD PRACTICE EXAMPLE 2.7

Care plan examples

George would like to have his subscription to *Gay Times* continued. He enjoys having some of the articles read out to him. He likes going through the 'personal ads' column thinking about who he might like to contact.

Rosaria would like to go out to a local gay pub with three of her closest female friends on a monthly basis.

(Knocker, 2006, p.28)

For those individuals who have/have had partners, validating those relationships is central to LGBTQ-affirmative care.

[It would] Be nice if you could have your partner's photo up, or have a place where you can be private together, or even, in a public place, hold hands without it being nudge-nudge wink-wink. *Doris, aged 69, lesbian* (Westwood, 2016b, p.1506)

Affirmative care is different from care that does not discriminate. Imagine that a new care worker goes into a straight woman's bedroom to help her get up and dressed. She sees a wedding photograph on the windowsill, and says, 'Oh, is that your husband? Isn't he handsome? Was that your wedding day? Oh, you both look so happy.' The next room she goes into is another older woman's. She has seen the woman's wife visit. Again, she sees a photograph on the windowsill, of the two of them on their wedding day. She says nothing. Now she has done nothing overtly wrong. She has said nothing bad or discriminatory. And she still gets the second woman up and dressed with equal care and kindness. But her silence speaks volumes, and conveys a powerful message. It is not a message of approval. And it is not affirmative care. What would have been affirmative care, would have been to say, as she had with the first woman, 'Oh, is that your wife? Isn't she lovely? Was that your wedding day? Oh, you both look so happy.'

GOOD PRACTICE EXAMPLE 2.8

Gloria is a 74-year-old Black woman of African Caribbean descent who lives independently in the community. Sonia (82 years), Gloria's partner of 40 years, has recently moved into a nursing home with a unit for adults with dementia. Gloria is not out to the care home staff but is extremely worried that a) the staff will restrict her from visiting her partner after hours and b) her partner has recently started chatting openly about their lives together with staff and telling other residents she's bisexual. Both Gloria and Sonia were in marriages with men in their early 20s before they met each other, and both identify as bisexual.

- What are Gloria's concerns here?

- What reassurance would you give to Gloria if Sonia was a resident in your home?

- How would you make both Gloria and Sonia feel welcome and valued?

- How would current policies in the care home support your responses?

- Are there any policies missing and how might you take this forward?

Top tips:

- Think of ways that the home can send clear messages to new residents and their loved ones about making everyone feel welcome and included. Producing a leaflet for partners of residents may help give some reassurances about equal treatment, respect and privacy for couples.

- Gloria may need to be reassured by a senior staff member or the manager that bisexual residents are welcome here and that she will be supported to spend time with her partner and be recognized as Sonia's partner.

- This might be a good time for rolling out some refresher training for all staff and managers on LGBTQ+ inclusion and equality. Part of the session could focus on the types of discrimination and challenges that bisexual people experience across their lifetime. It's important to recognize that LGBTQ+ people can experience different forms of discrimination and unequal treatment based on differences in gender, ethnic background and sexual identity.

- Some staff might hold stereotypical views about bisexual people that are not accurate or respectful; these need to be challenged.

> Care Under the Rainbow Case Studies (School for Policy Studies, University of Bristol and Diversity Trust, 2019, p.5)

Recognizing, and validating personal relationships, and including partners (if the person with dementia has a partner) and close friends and family in care and care decisions is central to LGBTQ+-affirmative care.

> The importance of inclusive residential aged care services was also highlighted by Jeremy (a gay man) who reported feeling socially isolated and depressed because he could not access the gay networks that were important to him. Whereas Tim described how a lack of privacy and concerns about homophobia made it difficult for him to spend time alone with his partner in residential aged care. (Barrett *et al.*, 2015, p.37)

Support for carers is vital too.

> Anne attended a carers' support service and reported 'a real warmth and camaraderie' with other carers that transcended sexual differences because they were all 'battling the same thing'. However, others like Richard felt 'a bit like a fish out of water' because the group was 'heteronormative', or focused on

heterosexual couples, and consequently he stopped attending. (Barrett *et al.*, 2015, p.37)

There are some examples of good practice, as can be seen below.

GOOD PRACTICE EXAMPLE 2.9

On one occasion...when I went into the small ward that he was in, one of the nurses said 'He's having his bath do you want to come in and help?'.... I mean, I'd been bathing him for months before, so why shouldn't I continue with that now? And they recognized that. Things like that really made us feel that we were being honoured and respected and accepted for who we were in relationship to each other. And so when he died and at that moment when he died and I always remember just pressing that buzzer and they came in and I remember the nurse saying 'You've just been wonderful.' Sorry. [Becomes tearful] It doesn't usually hit me like that, but she said 'You were there for each other.' And that's how it was.
Roger, gay man

(Social Care Institute for Excellence, 2011)

Conclusion

This chapter has highlighted the need to think differently about equality to meet the needs of LGBTQ+ people with dementia. While they share many issues and concerns with all people with dementia, there are specific issues relating to their sexualities and/or gender identities which need to be recognized, understood, respected and supported. Responding to their differences is essential for providing them with equally good care. Not all LGBTQ+ people are the same, and providing LGBTQ+ people with good dementia care does not require you to know everything about LGBTQ+ people before you work with them. It's impossible – because everyone is an individual, with their own separate histories and personalities and concerns. However, it does mean having a positive attitude towards working with LGBTQ+ people, and being open to learning from them. It means being willing to give them affirmative care – care that validates and celebrates LGBTQ+ people, rather than, at best, merely tolerating them.

FOOD FOR THOUGHT

- How can a member of staff do memory work with an LGBTQ+ person with dementia if they do not understand LGBTQ+ lives and histories?

- How can an LGBTQ+ person with dementia be supported in a memory group, if some of the other people in the group are homophobic or transphobic?

- Is it possible for a member of staff who disapproves of LGBTQ+ people, for example someone who thinks they are sinful and going to hell, to deliver LGBTQ+-affirmative care to someone with dementia?

- Bob, a man with dementia, married to a woman, has been admitted to a care home. He forms a romantic/sexual relationship with Sam, a widowed gay man who is also living in the home. Bob's wife says you must put a stop to it, as he was never 'like that' before dementia. Sam says Bob used to secretly meet men for sex, before he got dementia, without his wife ever knowing. What do you do?

KEY LEARNING POINTS

- ✓ Sometimes you have to treat people differently, to treat them equally well.

- ✓ Good practice with LGBTQ+ people with dementia involves recognition, understanding, respect and support.

- ✓ Recognition includes not assuming everyone is straight

or cisgender and creating environments and using language which are LGBTQ+ inclusive.

✓ Understanding involves appreciating the different ways in which LGBTQ+ people may have lived their lives, the challenges they have faced, and some still face, and appreciating what this means for dementia care.

✓ Respect goes beyond politeness. It involves valuing and celebrating each individual as human beings who have equal worth to all other human beings.

✓ Support for LGBTQ+ people with dementia must take into account the people, places, communities and activities that are important to them, and ensuring that these connections are maintained via robust care planning.

Chapter 3

Strategies for Good Practice in Dementia Care with LGBTQ+ People

---

Chapter summary

This chapter:

✓ invites you to think carefully about *taking a 'safe space' approach to delivering services*

✓ explains *what LGBTQ+-inclusive policies and procedures involve*

✓ outlines *relevant UK law and regulations*

✓ discusses *LGBTQ-affirmative care planning, LGBTQ+ staff inclusion*, staff recruitment, training and development

✓ discusses *LGBTQ+ community involvement* and *LGBTQ+ carer support*

✓ may be of particular interest to managers and organizational leaders.

Introduction

This chapter discusses the policies, procedures and strategies necessary to facilitate and maintain LGBTQ+-inclusive dementia care. We focus especially on recruitment, training and supervision and the importance of making sure all staff feel safe, confident and supported in dealing with LGBTQ+ issues. We highlight the importance of engaging with local LGBTQ+ communities in every aspect of dementia service provision. As in the previous chapters, we raise some questions at the end to help you think further about these issues.

A safe space approach

A safe space commitment sets out the expectations for everyone in a space – it forms an agreement for how people treat each other and what the space is like. As well as discouraging discriminatory behaviour, it helps to make LGBT people feel more confident that prejudice will be challenged. It also supports staff to do so in a firm but supportive way... It offers consistency and helps people to know what to expect, allows people to participate fully, and reduces uncertainties and anxiety. (LGBT Age, 2015, p.2)

LGBTQ+-inclusive dementia care involves creating environments where LGBTQ+ people feel safe to be openly themselves, and where their lives, life histories and relationships are validated, celebrated and affirmed. This safe space approach involves having LGBTQ+-inclusive policies and procedures, developing strategies to make sure LGBTQ+ staff feel safe and fully part of the team, and ensuring that staff recruitment and training promotes LGBTQ+ inclusion at all levels. It also means involving local LGBTQ+ groups and organizations in the design and delivery of care services.

It was such a relief when the manager of the extra care scheme where I was living encouraged me to open up about my lesbian identity. She didn't push me but she gave plenty of positive messages that she didn't have a problem. It immediately helped me to feel that I was accepted for the whole of me, and more important that I felt safe in my own home. *Anonymous quote* (Suffolk Lesbian, Gay, Bisexual and Transgender Network, 2012, p.6)

Policies and procedures
LGBTQ+-inclusive policies and procedures

> Policies and procedures can provide guidance for staff on what is expected of them in relation to LGBT people, helping them to make sure their practice is inclusive. (LGBT Health and Wellbeing, 2014, p.14)

Policies and procedures that are LGBTQ+-inclusive have the following characteristics (Westwood *et al.*, 2015; Hafford-Letchfield *et al.*, 2016):

1. They are written in a way which does not assume that staff, care recipients, their families and friends are heterosexual and/or cisgender.

2. All policies and procedures about residents' relationships are worded in such a way that they do not assume relationships are heterosexual and apply equally well to LGB and heterosexual people.

> It is the organization that needs to 'come out' as LGBT friendly rather than depending upon clients to 'come out' in order to get their needs met. (Age UK, 2017, p.32)

3. Equality and diversity policies make specific reference to LGBTQ+ rights in law.

4. There is a clear statement that the service/organization is LGBTQ+-inclusive and that prejudice or discrimination towards LGBTQ+ staff, service users, their families and friends will not be tolerated.

> It is important to understand that those of us who are members of minority groups are always looking for signs that we are 'included'. Failure to show such signs sends a message that our needs are neither considered nor met, and even, perhaps, that we are not welcome at all. *Roger Newman* (quoted in Switchboard, 2018, p.7)

5. There are procedures for how to deal with homophobia or transphobia committed by staff, service users, their families and friends. Staff are confident about how to challenge effectively and that they will be supported by their managers in doing so.

Policies and procedures also make LGBT people feel more confident and safer by reassuring them that they will be treated respectfully and protected from discrimination. (LGBT Health and Wellbeing, 2014, p.14)

6. Sexual orientation and gender identity are monitored (respecting confidentiality at all times). This avoids the assumptions that can sometimes be made that 'we don't have any LGBTQ+ people here' and can monitor improvements in the number of LGBTQ+ people who choose to be 'out' within the service.

7. There is guidance and support for staff with how to respond to:

- LGBTQ+ care users disclosing their sexualities/gender identities

- personal care issues affecting LGBTQ+ people

- gender identity issues for trans women and men experiencing memory loss

- performing memory work with LGBTQ+ people, some of whom may have complex relationship histories and/or may not feel comfortable exploring their life histories in groups with heterosexual and/or cisgender people.

Alice has never explicitly said this was a lesbian partnership... however, in respect to her story, the home has done a life story book, which includes many pictures and memories of the woman she shared her life with. Alice, who is now very frail, does not talk very much but still comes to life when her book is opened. (Age UK, 2017, p.32)

8. There is guidance for staff about using inclusive language with everyone. This includes not assuming that someone has/had a different sex partner or is heterosexual or cisgender.

9. There are strategies in place to explicitly welcome LGBTQ+ people to care services. Even small things, like the use of rainbow lanyards, can make a big difference, and convey a powerful message of inclusion. It is important that this is not done tokenistically, however. A rainbow lanyard worn in an organization that is not LGBTQ+-inclusive can be misleading to LGBTQ+ people.

When you discuss with clients, give them subtle messages to show that you are open to people of any sexual orientation or transgender identity. For example, you can do this by saying that you are a service provider which values diversity and is very inclusive towards your clients, no matter their gender identity, sexual orientation, race, disability or creed. (Suffolk Lesbian, Gay, Bisexual and Transgender Network, 2012, p.7)

10. Promotional materials are LGBTQ+-inclusive.

Promotional materials (brochures, leaflets, websites and so on)... should include visual representations of older LGBT people and should make explicit a service's commitment to working with older LGBT people. Healthcare, day care and residential establishments should have pictures and photographs representing older LGBT people, display LGBT publications and advice sheets, and hold LGBT social events and celebrations. (Westwood et al., 2015, p.149)

The first step in achieving LGBTQ+-inclusive policies and procedures is to audit what is already in place. Are the necessary policies and procedures in place? If so, how LGBTQ+-inclusive are they? What is missing? What needs to be improved to create greater LGBTQ+ inclusion? You may wish to use a checklist (see for example, Hafford-Letchfield et al., 2015 or Age UK, 2017). Sometimes it can be helpful to ask a local LGBTQ+ organization to assist you.

> There's a difference between those who say 'I'm here to tell you about diversity because they're making me do it to tick a box' and those who lead with conviction by saying 'I'm here to tell you about this because it's the right thing to do and I believe in it, and I want you to believe in it too, and these are the standards I expect. *Pam Hoey, straight LGBTQ+ ally* (quoted in Miles, 2011, p.30)

Once you have identified what needs to be done, you should develop new/revised materials (again, consulting with local groups can be useful), pilot them, see how they work, and fine-tune them if needed. It is also important to review all policies and procedures at least annually, to make sure they are still up to date, especially in relation to any new legal developments. You may also wish to do some further fine-tuning based on feedback from staff, people with dementia, their family and friends.

> Jim Glennon of Opening Doors London, a charity for older LGBT people, said that he would personally look for signs of inclusion if he were choosing a care home: 'People do not realize that, if we saw some marker and had confidence that this place, rather than that place, was doing the right things, with whatever, a sticker or a statement, we would choose to spend our money over there rather than over there. There is a business argument to be made.' (House of Commons Women and Equalities Committee, 2019, para 61)

Legal and regulatory requirements

> Everyone should have an equal opportunity to access high quality care and support to meet their individual needs and people should not be disadvantaged due to their background, culture or community. (Skills for Care, 2022, online)

It is essential that all policies and procedures are compliant with the law and with regulations. In the UK, the Equality Act 2010 prohibits discrimination, harassment and victimization against individuals on the basis of nine protected characteristics: age, disability, gender reassignment, marriage and civil partnership, pregnancy and maternity, race, religion or belief, sex, and sexual orientation.

The Care Act 2014 required local authorities and organizations acting on their behalf to deliver non-discriminatory services (Department of Health and Social Care, 2021, S 2.45). It requires personalized assessments and care planning (Barnes *et al.*, 2017).

> My partner got a letter saying, "'Home from hospital' will be taking over your care on Monday; it will be delivering services regardless of your sexual and gender orientation". We believe that practice should be stamped out. It is not appropriate to the Equality Act at all to say, "We will deliver a service regardless". The Care Act states it has to be personalized, and so does the Equality Act. *Dr Ju Gosling of Regard, an organization representing LGBT disabled people* (House of Commons Women and Equalities Committee, 2019, para 27)

The Care Quality Commission is committed to equality, diversity and human rights and has stated that 'there is growing evidence that equality and human rights for people using services and staff needs to play a central role in improving the quality of care' (Care Quality Commission, 2022).

> Discrimination is caused by a number of factors, including unconscious bias; stereotypical and prejudicial attitudes of staff; lack of specialist, cultural competence skills-based training; religious beliefs; cultural homophobia; lack of inclusive policies and procedures. All of these issues need to be addressed in order to create LGBT affirmative services. *Birmingham LGBT* (House of Commons Women and Equalities Committee, 2019, para 29)

The Human Rights Act 1998 incorporated the European Convention on Human Rights into UK law. Key articles under the convention which relate to care provision include: Article 2 (right to life); Article 3 (prohibition of torture and cruel, inhuman and degrading treatment); Article 5 (right to liberty and security); Article 8 (right to privacy and family life); Article 14 (prohibition of discrimination (in relation to the breach of other Articles).

Care planning

> Care and support is provided in accordance with people's preferences and personal histories. Staff respect people's wishes. (Care Quality Commission, 2019, p.10)

Strong, effective care planning is fundamental to personalized care for LGBTQ+ people living with dementia. As we explained in Chapter 2, it is essential that the needs, wishes, preferences and significant relationships of the LGBTQ+ person with dementia are fully included in their care plans.

> I certainly expect that my partner is treated equally with me, that we are part of a couple. I want that recognition that she's my next of kin and that she is the person that nursing staff talk to if I can't talk for myself or even if I can talk for myself and can't get it out very well. *Marie, 59-year-old lesbian* (Care Quality Commission, 2019, p.10)

Developing appropriate care plans for people with dementia should, first and foremost, include the person themselves, as well as those who know and understand them best of all.

> Ask for a contact person to whom information should be given, rather than using the term 'next of kin'...also find out the names of those people the patient wishes or does not wish to have contact with. (Royal College of Nursing, 2016, p.9)

Some LGBTQ+ people may have very good relationships with their family of origin, others may not, and may not wish them to be involved in their care. It is vital to understand who the important and trusted people are in the lives of each individual LGBTQ+ person living with dementia.

> As long as the people I want to associate with are permitted entry, and are accepted for who they are ... and aren't given any snide remarks or looks...then I'm happy with that. *John, aged 52, gay man* (King's College London ACCESSCare Research, 2017, p.9)

It is important for LGBTQ+ people and their visitors to be provided with privacy, so that they can be free and at ease with one another and not feel they have to be careful about what they say and do.

> Arrangements are made so people and visitors have appropriate space to spend time together, or for people to be alone. (Care Quality Commission, 2019, p.10)

It is important that the staff writing the care plans have sufficient knowledge, understanding and awareness of LGBTQ+ issues to be able to address them sensitively.

> Make sure all staff are appropriately trained so that they can talk openly about sexuality and gender, ask the right questions in a sensitive way and be aware of pronoun use. *Quote from a person with a non-binary identity* (Healthwatch, 2018, p.17)

Care plans only work if they are written properly, are regularly updated and all staff read and follow them.

> Sam is in their 70s and lives alone. Born into a male body, Sam spent much of their life feeling that something was wrong, and 20 years ago started to transition to female. They took hormones which made their breasts develop, but never had surgery to remove their male genitals. In recent years, Sam has started to identify as non-binary, and uses gender-neutral pronouns (they, them and their instead of he or she etc.).
> Sam developed dementia a couple of years ago, and the social work department arranged for support from a local provider. The social worker was aware of Sam's story, and informed the provider. However, Sam has now started to need personal care, and one of the support workers helping them with bathing screamed when she saw Sam's male genitals. Sam is now very anxious and unwilling to let anyone help with personal care. (LGBT Health and Wellbeing, 2020, p.12)

In this example, the problem stems from poor care planning.

The social worker told the care provider about Sam's story and so the care provider should have been aware of, and understood, the implications for Sam's general care, and if Sam was to ever need personal care. These issues should have been covered in a care plan, and discussed with Sam. All support workers should have read Sam's care plan, and they should have been supported in advance in terms of how best to provide Sam with personal care. There would then have been no shocks or surprises. This highlights the importance of staying on top of care planning and making sure that staff do too.

Becoming more LGBTQ+-inclusive

The following example shows what can be achieved by a provider when it decides to become more LGBTQ+-inclusive.

GOOD PRACTICE EXAMPLE 3.1

Anchor Hanover Housing recently piloted an LGBTQ+-inclusive housing scheme in Brighton. It implemented a coordinated programme of communication, marketing and learning and development, including:

- LGBTQ+ awareness training

- Marketing leaflet updated to include information relevant to LGBTQ+ residents, using more diverse images and reference to LGBTQ+ inclusion

- LGBTQ+ posters and leaflets on the scheme's noticeboards, and more diverse information in the scheme's newsletter

- LGBTQ+-inclusive and non-discrimination policies on all noticeboards

- Events organized to mark key dates (e.g. Pride events)

- Reviewing communal areas to ensure trans-inclusive signage

- Nurse practitioner at on-site surgery attending specialist LGBTQ+ training

- Engaging with local LGBTQ+ organizations, for example LGBTQ+ Switchboard, MindOut, The Clare Project and the Older and Out Project at Somerset Day Centre, Brighton.

According to Anchor Hanover, this was the impact:

- The percentage of residents identifying as LGBTQ+ doubled (from 5% to 10%).

- An 'increase in wellbeing' for all residents, including LGBTQ+ [residents]. 'We have completed Independent Living Outcomes to evaluate the changes.'

- Clear connections established with local LGBTQ+ organizations 'to be better equipped to signpost our residents to LGBT+-specific support'.

- 'Positive media coverage, including publicity in *Diva Magazine*.'

Anchor Hanover identified the following barriers, challenges and learning points:

- 'Inappropriate comments' from a resident 'resistant' to the promotion of LGBTQ+ services and events. 'Senior colleagues promptly met the resident to discuss acceptable behaviour so the issue didn't escalate. We have recently reviewed our ASB [anti-social behaviour] procedures which support this.'

- 'Colleague turnover. Refresher training put in place to ensure continuity of approach over time.'

- 'Ensuring consistent monitoring of sexual orientation, gender identity and trans status to adhere to best practice guidance.'

(National Housing Federation, 2022, online)

Anchor's initiative shows the creative ways a care provider can become more LGBTQ+-inclusive, and its benefits to LGBTQ+ service users and to its own reputation as a provider. It also highlights some of the challenges, including other service users who have negative attitudes towards LGBTQ+ people. The next chapter discusses ways to deal with these and other challenges.

Strategies

We will now discuss a range of strategies which promote LGBTQ+-inclusive care cultures.

LGBTQ+ staff inclusion

> LGBT staff need to be made to feel confident and comfortable in the workplace, by creating a culture of inclusion. If LGBT staff are comfortable at work it is much more likely that LGBT service users will be as well. (Westwood *et al.*, 2015, p.148)

LGBTQ+ staff can experience a lot of discrimination in the workplace. This can range from casual banter to hostile comments, homophobia and transphobia. These can come from colleagues, managers, service users or their families and friends.

> How can we possibly, as an organization, encourage our staff to give us all that they've got, without creating the right environment in which they can do that? We know that people perform better when they can be themselves – so how can you have an authentic relationship with colleagues if you don't feel that you can be yourself when you're at work? *Lucy Malarkey, straight LGBT ally* (quoted in Miles, 2011, p.28)

If LGBTQ+ staff are not confident and comfortable being open about themselves in the workplace, this will convey an unspoken message to LGBTQ+ service users, their families and friends. They will pick up on the fact that it is not safe to be 'out'.

These are the key ways to make sure LGBTQ+ staff feel safe at work (Jones-Schenk, 2018; Lim *et al.*, 2019; Ałabaster, 2022):

1. Ensure that all employment policies are fully and explicitly inclusive of LGBTQ+ rights, including in relation to relationship recognition, pregnancy and parenthood rights, pensions, health insurance, and so on.

2. If your organization is large enough, consider setting up an LGBTQ+ staff network. If it is not large enough to do so, try

connecting with other small organizations like your own, and set up a shared LGBTQ+ staff network instead.

3. Consult with LGBTQ+ employees about how they experience working in your organization, what works well for them, and what could be done better. Discuss any related changes with your LGBTQ+ employees before implementing them.

4. Consult with non-LGBTQ+ employees about both LGBTQ+ issues and non-LGBTQ+ issues, to make sure they do not feel that LGBTQ+ employees are being given special treatment in any way, and to make sure they are fully on board with addressing LGBTQ+ issues and resolving any problems.

5. Make sure that all staff – the most junior and the most senior – are fully engaged with creating an inclusive work environment for LGBTQ+ employees.

6. Monitor your staff for sexual orientation and gender identity, ensuring you treat their information with complete confidentiality and respect.

You get the best out of people if they're happy. If they feel afraid to be out, to talk openly or they feel they have to be careful about what they say or, even worse, if they fear 'banter' or discrimination – then they're not going to be happy and that will reflect on their work. So for me, as a manager, it's about making sure that your staff feel comfortable so they can be open about who they are. *Justine Williams, straight LGBT ally* (quoted in Miles, 2011, p.28)

Staff recruitment

Ensure at first stages of the recruitment process there are really rigorous and meaningful equality and diversity questions. To show you are truly inclusive you can add a statement when you advertise the vacancies that that you are open to LGBT clients. This is very likely also to deter people with prejudice...from applying. (Suffolk Lesbian, Gay, Bisexual and Transgender Network, 2012, p.10)

To ensure that you recruit staff who take a positive approach to working with LGBTQ+ people, it is important to set out your mission statements and values from the outset. That way people thinking about applying for your jobs will know from the start what kind of organization they will be working for, and whether they and your organization will be a good fit.

> **GOOD PRACTICE EXAMPLE 3.2**
>
> **Celebrating diversity, celebrating you**
> Anchor are committed to being a great and inclusive place to work. We want to hear from candidates from all backgrounds especially those who are from underrepresented groups. At Anchor, we live by the values of accountability, respect, courageousness and honesty and they go hand-in-hand with making sure we value diversity and champion an inclusive culture.
>
> We are a member of Inclusive Employers, a Stonewall Diversity Champion and a signatory to the Care Leaver Covenant and House-Proud Pledge schemes.
>
> (Anchor's website, 'Culture and Values' section, Anchor, 2022)

Staff training and development

> I think there needs to be more training of people in the dementia field...the LGBT community has unique needs. *LGBT person living with dementia* (Alzheimer's Association and SAGE Advocacy Services for LGBT Elders, undated, p.2)

Improving staff's knowledge and understanding will improve their practice with LGBTQ+ people with dementia.

> Understanding history...can enable service providers to better understand the experiences and perceptions that [LGBT] clients bring to their encounter with services. Hearing older [LGBT] people's narratives can highlight the historical context of inequality and oppression and is an important component of person- centred approaches. (Barrett *et al.*, 2016, p.105)

Good training will include the following (Westwood & Knocker, 2016; Higgins *et al.*, 2019):

- The wider historical context of LGBTQ+ people's lives.

- Diversity among LGBTQ+ people.

- Detailed and specific guidance on how to care for LGBTQ+ people with dementia, providing examples of good practice.

- The barriers faced by LGBTQ+ people, especially older LGBTQ+ people, in relation to accessing healthcare in general and dementia care in particular.

- A range of interactive activities and the opportunity for reflective discussion.

- Involving LGBTQ+ people in training design and delivery.

It is important that the training is delivered by skilled and experienced trainers, with expert knowledge about the issues affecting LGBTQ+ people with dementia. When choosing someone to provide such training, make sure to see their credentials. Ask to speak to other organizations similar to your own to find out how their training has been received elsewhere. As with anything else, shop around to make sure you are getting the right training package for your organization, delivered by people you feel you can work with.

> I feel this is one of the most difficult things we can come across in our work and I think we would all benefit from a training session, or several, to help us to better acknowledge the needs of trans individuals on receiving a diagnosis of dementia, and how these needs then change as the disease progresses. (quoted in Switchboard, 2018, p.42)

One-off training is generally not enough. There needs to be a rolling training programme, to make sure new staff benefit from the training and that staff who have previously attended get a refresher experience. The most effective training is implemented in parallel with a comprehensive review of policies, procedures and practices in your organization.

Online learning is also insufficient. It does not give staff the opportunity to fully explore the important issues, to voice concerns and, importantly, to reflect on their own personal attitudes and beliefs. There is a risk that online training can become merely a box-ticking exercise.

> A variety of experiential learning methods, including reflective exercises, video, role play, case studies and group discussion have the potential to enhance self-awareness, understanding and the sensitivity skills required to work effectively with older LGBT people. (Being Me Project, 2020, p.5)

It is very important that all staff, at all levels, involved in dementia care services undertake LGBTQ+ training, as each and every one of them contribute to the overall culture of a service.

> I think you've got to train right from the top, because you've got to get them, the senior management team, involved, because then it filters down, and then you can embed it in your policies, and you can ensure that your staff do what your policies set out you should do... It's not enough to have it sat in the policy book, is it? You have to use it. UK trainer (Westwood & Knocker 2016, p.42)

Some staff may have negative attitudes towards LGBTQ+ people. They need to be supported in reflecting on how those attitudes might affect their work and the quality of the service they deliver to LGBTQ+ people living with dementia, and to be made aware that they cannot express those negative attitudes at any time in the workplace.

> Health and social care learners are microcosms of wider society, thus they may have been socialized to hold heteronormative, heterosexist and homophobic/biphobic/transphobic attitudes towards older LGBT people. Educators need to support learners to understand how prejudices are formed and recognize the potential impact of their prejudices on the way they work with older LGBT people...[L]earners should be enabled to address their possible prejudices at both a cognitive and emotional level, and supported to

find positive means to address their prejudices. (Being Me Project, 2020, p.4)

This includes casual conversations with colleagues (who may themselves identify as LGBTQ+ or may be LGBTQ+ allies), which might be overheard and cause distress.

It affects everyone so it's important that straight people do pick up on inappropriate stuff they hear because that will really help gay colleagues that aren't out at work. They might leave work because there's a lot of homophobic 'banter' — so you could lose a good employee just because of stupid conversations in the office. *Alec Little, straight LGBT ally* (quoted in Miles, 2011, p.30)

Staff need to be helped to understand that unspoken disapproval can be sensed by LGBTQ+ people and will affect how safe they feel. They need to be helped to appreciate that care is not just about performing tasks, it is also about showing the person that you value them, and are interested in them, their lives and their relationships. Tolerance, if it involves simply 'putting up' with a person, is not enough.

I've had patients say to me, '… I'm pretty sure that other nurse doesn't like me very much.' … So, they have helped them to have a wash, they have helped them to get dressed or they have helped them with their medication and they have done everything, you know, appropriately, nothing untoward or wrong has happened, but they have basically ticked a list of tasks, they haven't actually provided care, that's the difference. And I think that's what the patients pick up on. *Claire, a nurse* (quoted in Westwood, James & Hafford-Letchfield, in press)

A study in the US has recently developed a checklist to determine whether staff are sufficiently skilled, informed and aware about LGBTQ+ issues to be able to effectively deliver services to LGBTQ+ people living with dementia (Nowaskie & Sewell, 2021). This may be helpful in supporting LGBTQ+ training, especially for evaluating its effectiveness.

Larger organizations may wish to develop their own training packages, while smaller organizations might want to work together to develop a shared one. It is important that this is done in collaboration with LGBTQ+ community organizations. LGBTQ+ members of staff should also be involved. However, it is important not to expect them to become the 'LGBTQ+ experts' on your service, especially as they will not necessarily know or understand the experiences of all people under the LGBTQ+ umbrella, especially those who are less like them.

> The biggest danger when you're looking for leadership is to find your most senior, open gay person and say 'because you're openly gay, and you're senior, you're now going to be the champion of LGB issues'. Why should that person be the champion of LGB issues just because they're openly gay? That's a real imposition. *Martin Hall, straight LGBT ally* (quoted in Miles, 2011, p.6)

Learning from experience

No one is perfect and we all make mistakes. Sometimes our learning is prompted by becoming aware of a situation where we need to do better, as the following good practice example shows.

GOOD PRACTICE EXAMPLE 3.3

Anna's Aunt Mary was being cared for in a nursing home. Anna was a regular visitor and well known to residents and staff. While Mary's health was deteriorating, Anna, after many years of internal struggle, had made the decision to undergo full gender reassignment... Anna told Mary she was undergoing treatment to become a woman. Mary responded positively to this news, so much so that when Anna visited subsequently, Mary would introduce her to other residents and staff as 'my new niece'... Many residents and staff would make comments once Anna had left, sometimes directly to Mary or indirectly, but still within earshot or sight. These hurtful remarks and ridicule left Mary feeling very distressed and were noticed by her carer who eventually spoke to Mary about it. Once the carer and social worker were aware of the situation they responded positively and spoke to Anna immediately to inform her of the insults and ridicule. The staff committed time to do some reading so they understood more about gender reassignment and the support Anna may need as she went through transition and cared for her aged aunt. Anna felt shocked and was devastated by the news, as it wasn't something she had expected, but she was also very impressed by the support and action of the staff. As intended, they did increase their understanding, the issue of ridicule and comment was addressed and stopped and Anna was consistently treated with respect. Sadly Mary died some while later when Anna was in hospital having her first operation, but she was comfortable, well cared for and content [that] the comments and ridicule had stopped. The whole experience has left Anna certain that she needs to be supported in a respectful way that accounts for her difference. Anna is also certain that if she ever needed to be cared for in a nursing home at the end of her life, then she would choose the same home as Aunt Mary.

(NHS National End of Life Care Programme, 2012, p.21)

This example shows how a bad situation can be turned into something good. Anna and Mary's negative experiences brought about cultural change, which resulted in improved services. This will have benefitted not only them, but also other care users and their carers from diverse backgrounds too.

LGBTQ+ community involvement

Involving LGBT+ people in shaping policies and practices on dementia care and taking a partnership approach between health, social care and the voluntary sector are all important in meeting the needs and hopes of LGBT people. (Social Care Institute for Excellence, 2020, online)

It is essential to include LGBTQ+ communities in your service design and development and to have regular and ongoing contact which supports creating LGBTQ+-inclusive environments. Some organizations now offer accreditation, which you may wish to consider (see the list of resources at the end of this book).

It's important for LGBT people to be around other LGBT people, as they share similar experiences. (Switchboard, 2018, p.75)

People are less likely to be seen as 'other' if they become part of everyday life. Perhaps local LGBTQ+ organizations could put on entertainment for the service users, their families and friends. Perhaps residents could be invited to LGBTQ+ events, such as Pride celebrations. LGBTQ+ inclusion benefits not only LGBTQ+ people living with dementia, but all those supporting people living with dementia.

The nasty comments didn't all stop straight away, of course, but after that delightful afternoon [with the LGBT choir] it was now other residents who joined in the rebuttals. (Age UK, 2017, p.32)

LGBTQ+ carer support

LGBTQ+ people living with dementia are not only those with memory loss but also LGBTQ+ carers supporting people with dementia, some of whom may not be LGBTQ+ themselves. LGBTQ+ carers can often feel lonely and isolated and have unmet support needs.

As an LGBTQ+ carer, I'd like to have been offered any info about any peer support communities (online or [in real life]) for LGBTQ+ carers of people with memory loss/dementia. (Switchboard, 2018, p.7)

It is important that dementia care providers ensure that LGBTQ+ carers are properly supported.

Mum's attitudes have gone back in time as her memory has failed so she can be homophobic and transphobic which is painful even though I know she can't help it. She forgets to use my chosen name rather than my birth name. I either have to keep coming out to the ongoing stream of new professionals involved in her care or be assumed to be straight and monogamous – it's a bit exhausting. (Switchboard, 2018, p.75)

It is important that the support on offer is itself LGBTQ+-inclusive.

It is no good directing an LGBTQ+ carer to a carer support group if it does not welcome them. It could make them feel even more isolated if some of the people in the group are uncomfortable around LGBTQ+ people and/or have negative attitudes towards them.

> I don't feel that my commitments to my family of choice are as recognized or as valued as a conventional heterosexual monogamous marriage would be. Because Mum, the person I care for, is heterosexual I feel like I am torn between two worlds. I want to support her to remain as active as possible in her community. But I also want to have the time and energy left to engage with my own community. (Switchboard, 2018, p.75)

Setting and auditing standards

CELEBRATE YOUR SUCCESSES

> Making sure your organization is LGBT-inclusive is an ongoing journey, so it's important to celebrate your successes, whatever size they may be, along the way. Every step is a step towards acceptance without exception for LGBT people. (Alabaster, 2022, online)

Policies and procedures only work if they are properly implemented. It is important to set standards and then to routinely monitor and audit them to make sure they are being maintained. Using a checklist can be helpful in conducting an audit (this one may be of use, see Gay & Lesbian Health Victoria (GLHV), 2016, pp.4–9). In particular, it is important to look for LGBT+-inclusive practice standards; ongoing LGBTQ+-inclusive programme development; LGBTQ+ staff support; LGBTQ+-inclusive workforce recruitment, staff supervision and training; quality controls and service reviews; LGBTQ+-inclusive care planning; LGBTQ+ carer support; and strategies to respond to LGBTQ+ prejudice and discrimination by staff, volunteers, service users and/or their families and friends.

> One of the lovely things for us is that, by word of mouth, we now

have a great reputation for being a very gay-friendly service. (Age UK, 2017, p.32)

Conclusion

This chapter has highlighted how LGBTQ+ inclusion underpins every aspect of dementia care, including an organization's policies, procedures and strategies. They all contribute to establishing an organization's core values and informing its culture. Policies, procedures and strategies will not change staff attitudes, but they will make sure staff are knowledgeable about LGBTQ+ issues. They will also encourage staff development that is underpinned by the principles of equality, diversity and inclusion. They will ensure that staff know how to challenge unacceptable language and behaviour (more on this in the next chapter) and are confident that they are supported by their managers in doing so. When implemented properly, the right policies, procedures and strategies will create a safe space for LGBTQ+ people to work in, receive dementia care, and be supported as carers.

GOOD PRACTICE EXAMPLE 3.5

The charity Dementia Support

At Dementia Support we want to help everybody live well with dementia. We work tirelessly to improve the support we offer; this includes educating ourselves and working in partnership with organizations more knowledgeable than ourselves, like Chichester Pride and the LGBT Foundation. That's also why some of our staff undertook the LGBT Champions training and have shared what they learnt with the rest of the team.

We know it's a journey, much like dementia, to keep ourselves educated and responsible for being a strong advocate for members of the LGBTQ+ community living with dementia, but we will keep working on it.

(Dementia Support, 2022, online)

FOOD FOR THOUGHT

- How do you balance the pressures of covering shifts, and the need to use bank/agency staff at times, with making sure those bank/agency staff are adequately trained and skilled in supporting LGBTQ+ people with dementia?

- How can you ensure that all your staff have regular ongoing training on LGBTQ+ issues, especially if you have a high staff turnover?

- Are your policies, procedures and strategies LGBTQ+-inclusive? If not, what are you going to do to address this?

- How do you currently audit your policies, procedures and strategies for LGBTQ+ inclusiveness? Does this need to change?

- Have you explored your own knowledge and understanding of LGBTQ+ issues, and attitudes towards LGBTQ+ people? Do you have any blind spots? If so, how are you going to address them?

KEY LEARNING POINTS

✓ Safe spaces are where people can openly be themselves, including LGBTQ+ people living with dementia.

✓ LGBTQ+-inclusive policies and procedures let staff, LGBTQ+ people living with dementia and their families and friends know where they stand and what standards are expected of everyone.

✓ Making sure LGBTQ+ staff feel safe to be open at work will encourage LGBTQ+ people living with dementia, and LGBTQ+ people supporting loved ones with dementia to be open too.

✓ Making LGBTQ+ inclusion explicit in all staff recruitment will encourage staff to apply who have positive attitudes towards LGBTQ+ people.

✓ Ongoing staff training and development regarding LGBTQ+ issues, linked to performance management, will encourage LGBTQ+-inclusive practice.

✓ Delivering services to LGBTQ+ people living with dementia involves supporting not only LGBTQ+ people who have dementia, but also LGBTQ+ people who are informal carers to people with dementia.

✓ Creating and maintaining ongoing relationships with local LGBTQ+ organizations and involving them in all aspects of your service will ensure that it is ready to welcome LGBTQ+ people living with dementia, and that you have established connections you can turn to for guidance and support when needed.

Chapter 4

Dealing with Challenges

Chapter summary

This chapter:

- ✓ considers some of the *key challenges associated with delivering services to LGBTQ+ people living with dementia*

- ✓ suggests some *strategies for how to overcome them*

- ✓ discusses *how to engage with staff who disapprove of LGBTQ+ people in ways which may influence the quality of the care they provide*

- ✓ addresses *how to respond to other people with dementia who disapprove of LGBTQ+ people* and express this in hurtful ways

- ✓ explores *how to deal with the families and friends of people with dementia who are prejudiced and/or discriminatory towards LGBTQ+ people with dementia* in your care and/or their friends and families

- ✓ identifies the *importance of staff feeling confident and supported in challenging prejudice and/or discrimination*, including in relation to LGBTQ+ issues.

Introduction

This chapter explores some of the key challenges that can arise when delivering care to LGBTQ+ people with dementia, including in relation to staff, service users, their families and friends. It also considers what to do when LGBTQ+ people with dementia need you to advocate for them. We provide detailed case studies in this chapter, to give you lots of opportunity to see how specific challenges can be dealt with in practice. Each of the case studies raises certain questions, which we suggest you might wish to reflect on. First, we discuss ways to constructively challenge inappropriate or offensive behaviour.

How to challenge constructively

> When I met my husband he was sexist, racist, homophobic – every 'ism' you can think of. But eighteen months ago he was on a float at Pride. I've challenged him, I've challenged his friends – and I use him as an example to talk about how attitudes can be changed. Colleagues find it amusing but it gets the point across that if he can do it, anybody can. *Elaine Prescott, straight LGBT ally* (quoted in Miles, 2011, p.30)

We all need to be able to let someone know if they have behaved in ways they should not have done, and to do so in a manner which makes it most likely they will be able to hear what it is we have to say.

GOOD PRACTICE EXAMPLE 4.1

Yeah we had a patient a couple of months back...it never occurred to me that he was gay. But somebody pointed it out and said – oh there's his boyfriend...and everybody just took the mick out of him and one caregiver did openly say – 'well he's a gay boy' – and he was next to the station so he would have heard it. And so I had to take him out and you know ask him to apologize. *Joan (District nurse) North West*

(Hunt, Cowan & Chamberlain, 2007, p.27)

At the heart of challenging someone is assertiveness – clearly and effectively communicating your thoughts, wants and needs. Some of us can find it quite hard to be assertive, perhaps because we lack confidence, or we don't want to upset others, or because we fear we might become angry and aggressive. However, assertiveness is important for open and honest communication, which is essential in all walks of life, but especially when working in the care sector, where colleagues and people using services deserve honesty and transparency. If people do not know they are behaving in ways which make you feel uncomfortable, then they will not have the opportunity to do something about it. Assertiveness is also needed when responding to criticism. No one is perfect. We all have areas where we need to improve. Receiving criticism as constructive feedback, rather than an attack, is a mark of maturity and professionalism.

> **Assertive people are able to be honest about their thoughts and feelings in a respectful way. They actively listen to and are considerate of other people's perspectives. Assertive people are able to maintain control over their feelings and admit when they've made a mistake. (Psychology Today 2022, online)**

When speaking to someone – whether it is a colleague, manager, person with dementia, their family or friends, other visitors – about something they have said and done, it is important not to put them on the defensive. Make sure you speak to the person in private, at a time when they are not distracted, and in a place where you cannot be overheard (to respect their privacy). Be clear and precise, focus on what it is they have said and done, rather than who they are as a person. Empathize. Offer solutions. Make sure they have a way out of the situation and can save face. Stay calm, do not use abusive language and don't make threats. Do not apologize.

CHALLENGING THE BEHAVIOUR NOT THE PERSON

When dealing with a tricky situation, remember to explain clearly what the problem with the behaviour is, and explain how they might change it. While they should take responsibility for their actions, it's important not to characterize them as a bad person – they may

not have realized that what they were doing was hurtful, and challenging them gently but firmly is the most effective way to support them to change their behaviour. If someone does have a prejudiced opinion, and isn't willing to change it, you can take the line that regardless of their views, it's not acceptable to express prejudice in the space. (LGBT Age, 2015, p.2)

There are some phrases which can be helpful to use (see the box below). Some of you reading this book may recognize them as phrases that you already use. Some of you may see some phrases you may want to try in the future. Some of you might think you cannot imagine yourself speaking in that way. But you would be surprised how quickly, with practice, they can become part of how you communicate, and how effective they can be.

SOME USEFUL PHRASES

- 'I need to remind you that it is important we speak to and about each other in respectful ways at all times.'

- 'May I remind you that we have all made a commitment to ensuring that this is a safe and welcoming space for everyone.'

- 'It's important that we think about how our words might affect others, isn't it? I wonder how you might feel if someone spoke like that about you?'

- 'Can I just stop you there. The language you are using is not appropriate. Please speak about other people with respect.'

- 'It is essential that we use the right pronouns for a person at all times, whether or not they can hear us. Please use "she" and "her" (or "he" and "his") when talking about X.'

- 'You seem to be making assumptions here. Where is your evidence to support what you are saying?'

- 'Please don't use that word/those words as they are very offensive.'

- 'I understand that these are your personal beliefs, but they do not belong in the workplace.'

- 'We do not discriminate here.'

(Adapted from multiple sources)

You will see the term 'straight ally' used a lot in this chapter. A straight ally is someone who does not themselves identify as LGBTQ+ but speaks out about LGBTQ+ rights.

> **When lesbian or gay colleagues get up and talk about LGBT issues, people hearing those issues may say 'well you would say that, wouldn't you – because you're a member of the gay community'. When straight allies say the same thing, it has a different impact.**
> **Chris Murray, straight LGBT ally** (quoted in Miles, 2011, p.5)

LGBTQ+ people living with dementia have the right to enjoy their lives with dignity and respect. LGBTQ+ staff and LGBTQ+ families and friends deserve to be valued, included and supported just like anyone else. They all deserve to feel safe. Everyone – LGBTQ+ people and non-LGBTQ+ people – should play a part in that.

Sometimes LGBTQ+ staff and/or their LGBTQ+ allies have to deal with homophobic and/or transphobic abuse directed at themselves. This needs to be challenged constructively. The following good practice example shows how care organizations can provide structured guidance and have procedures for how to respond.

GOOD PRACTICE EXAMPLE 4.2

How to respond to abusive behaviour

- Being on the receiving end of abusive behaviour, especially if it involves prejudice and discrimination, can be extremely difficult for service users and members of staff. It is important that staff do not retaliate, both because they need to maintain professional standards, and because it would only escalate things.

- The service should make clear to service users, and to visitors, that abuse will not be tolerated.

- All incidents of abusive behaviour should be recorded, investigated, and the actions taken also placed on record. Possible actions might include:

  o A conversation with the person who has been abusive, explaining that their behaviour is not acceptable.

  o A written warning.

  o In the case of visitors, monitored visits, and, as a last resort, and only in consultation with expert advisors and regulators, the possibility of prohibited visits.

  o In the case of the person who has been abusive lacking the capacity for insight (e.g. if this is a service user with severe dementia symptoms) for a care plan to be devised with strategies to minimize the risk of further abuse, and manage incidents accordingly.

- Staff should be supported, via training and supervision, to develop ways of responding to verbal abuse assertively and constructively.

- Staff who have experienced verbal and/or physical abuse should be provided with support at the time of an incident, and also following on from it as well.

- It is important to explore whether there are any issues relating to a person's condition and/or care which may have contributed to the abuse, and to adapt care delivery where appropriate.

(Adapted from multiple sources)

Staff who resist LGBTQ+ inclusion

> I genuinely don't believe that the vast majority of nurses and health-care support workers get up and go to a shift with the intention of deliberately discriminating against LGBT communities. What they may well experience is the impact of unconscious bias. *Wendy Irwin from the Royal College of Nursing* (quoted in House of Commons Women and Equalities Committee, 2019, para 30)

While many colleagues will be in full agreement with delivering LGBTQ+-inclusive services, this may not always be the case. It is important that staff who are not fully committed to LGBTQ+ inclusion are helped to understand an organization's core values and that they must work with, and fully support them, in order to work effectively for the organization. This should also be addressed through their supervision and professional development.

GOOD PRACTICE EXAMPLE 4.3

Some staff had strong views about our Safe Zone LGB training – why was it being done and did they have to participate? I made it very clear that this is training that all staff undertake and explained the reasons why – it's about ensuring that everybody's treated fairly and that people feel comfortable in the workplace. I also made it very clear that this is how we expect people to behave when they're in the workplace. *Justine Williams, straight LGBT ally*

(Miles, 2011, p.30)

Sometimes, people may make casual throwaway remarks without realizing the hurt they can cause. It is important that this is challenged, as can be seen from the following good practice example.

GOOD PRACTICE EXAMPLE 4.4

A lot of people will say 'that's so gay' and I don't allow that to happen. I take that person away and I talk to them about it. I explain why it isn't acceptable – that there are gay people who work here and they're not going to find that funny. I'm aware all the time of what they're saying and they're aware of the boundaries now – you can see a real difference in the way that they're with people. *Wendy Lister, straight LGBT ally*

(Miles, 2011, p.30)

People often say 'I was only joking' when challenged about a homophobic or transphobic comment. But jokes hurt. They can cause pain and distress to LGBTQ+ colleagues, to LGBTQ+ people with dementia, to their families and friends (who may or may not identify as LGBTQ+ themselves) and to straight allies of LGBTQ+ people. If such jokes go unchallenged this can form part of a culture that is not fully LGBTQ+-inclusive.

> Members of my family are gay – they're not an alien race. They're my closest family members in every way. I'd stick up for my sister if she was being picked on. I don't think about it. I just do it because you believe in it. I don't go out of my way to be a guardian of gay rights – that's not what it's about. It's just instinctive. *Martin, straight LGBT ally* (quoted in Miles, 2011, p.30)

Of course, on occasions some colleagues and managers can be overtly hostile towards LGBTQ+ people. They may speak to or about them in ways that are not acceptable. This must be constructively challenged.

> Speak up! If you see or hear any transphobic bullying or misgendering, speak up in support of your trans co-workers and be prepared to report things to line managers if need be. Let other colleagues know that a trans person's name or pronouns have changed if you notice this is happening. (Trades Union Congress, 2019, p.8)

LGBTQ+ people living with dementia often receive very good care and support, as the following example shows. However, the example also raises a few questions as well.

GOOD PRACTICE EXAMPLE 4.5

Greg and Kevin: It's there in front of you

Greg (diagnosed with dementia): It's been frustrating. I get halfway through the conversation if it is interesting, and I lose the focus on it. You don't stop being gay if you get dementia...being gay is part of your life, a part of your make-up. No, we can't make being gay disappear, it's there in front of you.

Kevin: Greg and I have been together for nearly 40 years. I'm 75. We have never been the type to flaunt our sexuality. If anybody asks, yes, they're told... We have quite a few lesbian neighbours, we look after them, they look after us... I think it's important to mix with gay people because...when you're mixing with your own type, if you like, you speak freer.

Greg's been assessed and we have a case manager who organizes things and rings up regularly to see if I'm okay... We've got a package of care... Greg and I have a respite day twice a week and he is picked up from home by taxi, driven to the respite house; he goes to that with a group of people. He's brought home at about three o'clock so I have that day to myself... Later in the week he's picked up by taxi and taken out to their day centre and then brought home again late afternoon. A cleaner comes... It's normally the same lady...but there are the odd times when I've had to cancel and try and get another day. It's obvious to whoever comes to work through the house that Greg and I are sleeping in the same bed and all that. No questions asked, no problem, they joke with us, good with us, no problem at all.

It was interesting, our case manager we've had for quite a while – I took it for granted that she's put two and two together. Months ago, something came up, and I said, 'You're obviously aware that Greg and I are gay,' and she said then, 'No, I wasn't.' She said to me, 'Well, when I first met you two it never entered my head that you might be gay.' She was fine with it. She's also got somebody else who is gay I think, and I also know our home help lady has had to actually do cleaning for friends of ours who are gay.

(Crameri *et al.*, 2015, pp.14–15)

Greg is clear that being gay does not diminish with dementia.

Kevin describes receiving a good service, which supports both Greg and himself. He and Greg experience warm acceptance and inclusion. Their care and support go beyond tasks being performed to them but being performed in a friendly, human way, with humour, by staff to whom it is clear that Greg and Kevin are long-term partners. All this is to be celebrated.

However, there are some points of concern. Kevin describes not 'flaunting' their sexuality, suggesting that they feel the need to conceal it at times. This is understandable. There are many places and spaces where it is still not safe to be openly gay. And for Greg and Kevin, who spent much of their adult lives against a background of same-sex sexualities being criminalized, the need to conceal is deeply ingrained. Greg's dementia has undermined their ability to conceal, however. The need for care and support means that Greg and Kevin's life together is now much more on show than it was before.

Kevin had assumed that their care manager knew that he and Greg were gay. It came as a shock to him to find out that she did not know. Her not knowing means that none of her own care and support, Greg's care plan, or the respite and day care, was designed with the needs of a gay man in mind. This sexuality-blind provision may not seem problematic on the surface, given that Greg and Kevin are receiving good care, but on closer inspection it is.

As this book has explained, treating everyone the same is not enough to provide individualized, personalized care. As Kevin has said, he and Greg feel freer when they are mixing with other gay/lesbian people. So, their support package should have taken this into account. Would Greg have preferred to go to respite/day care with other LGBTQ+ people, for example? Would Kevin like to be connected with other LGBTQ+ dementia carers?

It will make you feel more isolated if you're treated as straight or if you're treated as peculiar if you're not straight. *Iris, lesbian, aged 61, living in sheltered accommodation* (Westwood, 2016a, p.e157)

It is to be hoped that the case manager reflects on not seeing what was 'there in front of' her. She may wish to ask herself why she did not explore sexual orientation and gender identity in her assessments and her care planning with Greg and Kevin. She may wish to explore her assumptions and consider what they mean for her practice. She may identify some professional development and learning needs. Sometimes it is not others we need to challenge to do better, it is ourselves.

Religious and cultural tensions

> One older disabled lesbian woman describes being given leaflets by religious care workers suggesting that she could be 'saved'; an experience that has made her feel unsafe and alienated in her own home. (Knocker, 2012, p.10)

Some LGBTQ+ people are people of faith, and many religious individuals and organizations are inclusive of LGBTQ+ people. However, some religious people disapprove of LGBTQ+ people and disagree with their rights, such as same-sex marriage. Some even think LGBTQ+ people are going to Hell. This includes some religious care providers (Westwood, 2022a).

> 'As a lesbian I would be worried that there would be discrimination by staff with a religious based anti-gay ethos.'
>
> 'Care providers with strong religious convictions such as homosexuality is sinful may treat LGBT people with less respect and dignity than they should.'
>
> 'A lot of religions are homophobic/transphobic and don't respect the rights of LGBTQ+ people. This can lead to religious individuals being homophobic/transphobic when required to provide care for LGBTQ+ people.'
>
> *Statements by LGBTQ+ participants in a recent UK research project on religion, sexuality and gender identity in older age care* (Westwood, 2022b, p.13)

There have been reports from researchers in the UK who have

encountered care staff holding very strong negative views about LGBQT+ people.

> One staff member declared...that they 'knew how to deal with that disease' and 'one woman [care staff member] stated she would ban her son from the house if he came out as gay. (Hafford-Letchfield et al., 2018, p.e318)

There have also been reports from people in the UK delivering LGBTQ+ training to health and social care staff who have come across deeply held religious prejudice towards LGBTQ+ people. Sometimes this had led to those staff refusing to engage in the training, or attending the training if it was mandatory, but only 'going through the motions' when there.

> One woman said that if her daughter was lesbian she'd have to 'exorcize the demon out of her' and another man just starting from the point of 'where does this perversion come from?' on the training and then wanting to go into the whole spiel about how the male and female anatomy are meant for each other. Joy, UK trainer (Westwood & Knocker, 2016, p.18)

Even though these attitudes and beliefs will be deeply offensive to many people, it is important that they are heard so that they can be discussed and explored, particularly in terms of how they may affect a person's practice.

> It can be hard...you know one guy came in and said, 'what causes this perversion?' and I've been prayed over, and there's been this uprising in the room with people saying, 'Oh if my daughter was...' and all this gay conversion stuff, and it's been pretty, pretty tough, yeah. But...you've got to hear the hatred, actually, and sort of expose it, rather than it just staying as subtext. Sarah, UK activist trainer (Westwood & Knocker, 2016, p.18)

People are entitled to their religious beliefs. Those beliefs are, however, a private matter. They should not be brought into the workplace, and they should in no way inform how care is delivered to an LGBTQ+ person living with dementia.

> We need to be doing more experiential training. They need to have a chance to place themselves in a different situation, get personally involved and challenge their way of thinking. I think people can shift attitudes if you approach it in the right way. You need to draw people out and hear their prejudices and they need to hear what you have to say. *Roger, older gay man* (Knocker, 2012, p.18)

Allowing one's religious beliefs to affect the quality of care being delivered is contrary to equality law and to professional regulations. Recently, in the UK, a hospital doctor was dismissed for refusing to use the correct pronouns with trans patients, on the grounds of his religious beliefs; a psychotherapist was struck off for engaging in religious-based conversion therapy; and a nurse lost her job after repeatedly preaching at patients and interrogating them about their religious beliefs. However, making sure our religious beliefs do not affect our practice with LGBTQ+ people goes beyond these extreme examples. It is important that care providers can, hand on heart, authentically provide affirmative care to LGBTQ+ people living with dementia. They must approve of, and accept, LGBTQ+ people as much as they would anyone else. Care providers must be able to celebrate LGBTQ+ lives and their relationships, past and present. If a person's religious beliefs prevent them from doing so, this is something they and their managers must address.

> I think as managers it's not just about managing work, it should be about influencing people too. You still work with lots of people whose perceptions have never been challenged – but through education and by discussing issues when they happen, you can really see their behaviour changing. As a manager, I feel I'm in a good position to do that within my team. *Wendy Lister, straight LGBT ally* (quoted in Miles, 2011, p.28)

Sometimes it can be challenging for care staff who come from overseas, from countries where LGBTQ+ people are criminalized and/or regarded as mentally ill, to adjust to LGBTQ+ social and legal acceptance in the UK. It can take time, and education, to help them adjust their perspectives. They are entitled to all the help and support they need in doing so.

> ...support workers who come from abroad...from countries where [LGBT people] face a criminal offence, punishment by death, come to a country where it's very accepted ... they go on a journey trying to get their head around it because they come from a country where they're supposed to really, really hate people to a country where they accept gay people. *Farid* (Peel & McDaid, 2015, p.14)

It is important that everyone in the team takes responsibility for any negative attitudes or behaviour towards LGBTQ+ people, whether informed by religion or otherwise.

GOOD PRACTICE EXAMPLE 4.6

Clare describes challenging a religious nurse who had just told a gay patient that she would pray for him.

> And then I caught her, because she was at the meds trolley and went, 'Look, I just want to ask, what did you mean when you said you'd pray for him?' I think she was in her early 40s... And then she went, 'Oh, no it was because he's a gay, he's going to go to Hell.'... I said, 'I understand that you have, you know, deep-seated religious beliefs, that you believe that is the case, but you can't express it to patients, that's not acceptable, because you are basically disapproving of their life and that's not good.'... Well, she looked at me, I don't think anyone has ever called her on it before, she sort of looked at me sideways and went, 'Well, I'll pray for you too.' *Claire, a nurse* (quoted in Westwood, James & Hafford-Letchfield, in press)

The example shows how to challenge someone respectfully. The nurses' religious beliefs are acknowledged and not criticized. At the same time, the non-acceptability of expressing those beliefs was also made clear. No doubt Clare informed her manager, who would, ideally, have followed this up in supervision and via performance management. As can also be seen from the example, challenging someone, however constructively, does not produce immediate change. It is all part of a process, which will hopefully lead to change in the longer term.

Service users with negative attitudes towards LGBTQ+ people

People with dementia can be prejudiced, just as much as people without dementia can be. Sometimes that prejudice is exposed in their language more than it would have been before they had dementia, because it has made them more disinhibited. They may also lash out more verbally because they are confused, frightened and frustrated. Challenging someone with dementia can be difficult, partly because they may not understand and partly because they may not remember. However, it is still important that they are challenged, because care teams, and carers, need to maintain standards for appropriate speech and behaviour.

> My father had dementia, and I was his sole carer until he died. He was white (as am I), born in England in the 1920s and used lots of the colloquial terms of a Londoner from that time. Some of those terms referred to Black people, some of them celebratory, some of them not. When his dementia was fairly progressed, he was in hospital occasionally due to falls, and while we were there he would make comments about the Black nurses. In his mind, he was paying them compliments, about them being hard-working, but the language he used did not convey this. At this point he had trouble remembering the end of a sentence and so he could not remember being told not to speak that way. Even so, every time he used an offensive word, I would gently say, loudly enough so that the other patients and staff could hear, 'I know you mean no offence, but that language is not acceptable.' It made no difference to him, but I hoped it would make a difference to those people who might overhear him and be offended. It also made a difference to me because I needed to make clear that the language he was using was not language I supported. *Sue (co-author), lesbian*

GOOD PRACTICE EXAMPLE 4.7

We found that after we took a stronger approach as a staff team when Mrs H made comments about 'those awful queers', some of the other day centre members used to tick her off too.

(Age UK, 2017, p.32)

Sometimes, negative attitudes go beyond the occasional inappropriate use of language and involve wider scale exclusions. The following good practice example shows how this was dealt with by a day centre.

GOOD PRACTICE EXAMPLE 4.8

Pat's story (day care)

Pat is a 73-year-old transgender male who has had a diagnosis of dementia for five years. He lives with his partner of 35 years who is finding it difficult to care for him and feels that a few days of day care would benefit them both.

Pat and his partner came to view the Day Centre and were both impressed with the surroundings, meals and daily activities on offer. However, Pat's partner was nervous about how Pat would be received by staff. Pat's partner was reassured by the Manager and it was agreed that Pat would come for day care two days a week.

On day one, other members at the centre commented on Pat's appearance/looks and behaviours and some staff 'giggled' at these without showing concern for Pat and his feelings.

After the third week Pat's partner spoke to the Manager and stated that Pat was getting upset on the days he was due to attend day care. Pat came home from day care upset and agitated. He felt that he was being ignored, laughed at and excluded from activities.

The Manager agreed to observe the situation when Pat was next in the centre. He observed that Pat seemed to sit at a table on his own for meals and he wondered why Pat was not always invited to participate in games and activities when he could participate.

The Manager spoke to staff regarding Pat's time in the centre and explained that Pat's partner had identified some issues of concern.

The Manager organized to speak with staff and planned a training and development programme for them, focusing on sexual identity and orientations, human rights, diversity and respect for personhood.

(Health and Social Care Board, 2020, p.7)

It is not clear from this example how effective the manager's interventions were. It also concerning that he had not already picked up on the way Pat was being mocked and excluded, and how he was socially isolated at meals – especially since Pat's partner had shared concerns from the outset. It is to be hoped that staff and day centre service users became more tolerant and inclusive towards Pat. This would need to be monitored on an ongoing basis, and risk assessed in relation to Pat's care and wellbeing while at the day centre.

Friends and family of service users with negative attitudes towards LGBTQ+ people

Challenging a person with dementia's friends and family can be a daunting prospect. Supporting someone with dementia can be stressful for their family and friends and sometimes their sense of loss, grief, sadness and frustration can lead to them saying and doing things that cause offence.

Care providers have a duty to ensure their services are safe for all, including LGBTQ+ people. Inappropriate language or behaviour cannot be tolerated. Having a policy which makes this clear, displaying it in public places, and giving a copy of it to all new visitors, will help to set boundaries. If a visitor speaks or behaves inappropriately to or about LGBTQ+ people, then they should be constructively challenged, in the ways outlined at the beginning of the chapter. If they do so repeatedly, then strategies need to be put in place to manage their visits.

Sometimes, when someone enters a care home it can expose long-standing family divisions, which need to be handled carefully. In the case of LGBTQ+ people living with dementia, there can be tensions between a person with dementia's family of origin and their partners, family and friends. These tensions can become heightened when the biological family members do not accept or respect the LGBTQ+ person with dementia's sexuality and/or gender identity.

> Many health care professionals will only discuss a patient's issues with the 'next of kin'. This is often unofficially presumed to mean a blood relative or heterosexual spouse. For day to day care of clients without a registered partner or spouse, the patient's or client's wishes in their choice of nominated person should be respected. With regard to matters of consent to treatment for those unable to freely provide it, you should seek advice from your employers. The underlying rule must be to always act in the patient's best interest. (Royal College of Nursing, 2016, p.4)

This is one of the reasons it is so important to make sure, where at all possible, that the person with dementia nominates the person they want to be their representative (also known as 'next of kin'). It is also why making advance directives and assigning powers of attorney are so important for LGBTQ+ people. That way they can make sure that the people they want to be involved in their lives are, and that the people they do not want to be involved are not.

When tensions do arise, it is important to deal sensitively with them, as the following example shows.

GOOD PRACTICE EXAMPLE 4.9

Collette and Roisin's story (care home)

Roisin and Collette had lived together as a couple for several years. When Collette received a diagnosis of Alzheimer's disease, Roisin cared for her at home for almost two years before her own health deteriorated and she found herself no longer able to cope with the physical demands of caring. They spoke to the Social Worker and agreed that the additional care which Collette needed could best be met in a Care Home.

After Collette moved into the Home, Roisin visited frequently and Collette looked forward to these visits. She and Roisin would sit together and hold hands and were able to enjoy more intimate time together in Collette's room.

Collette's family were never happy about the relationship and felt that because Collette was more vulnerable and being cared for by staff at the Home, staff should refuse Roisin admission to the Home and certainly not allow her to be alone with Collette in her room.

The Home Manager spoke to relatives about the Home's safeguarding policy and explained that consideration had been given to Collette's past history and her relationship with Roisin. She explained too that staff would always be vigilant to signs of distress during visits and through assessments by the Dementia Specialist, it had been established that Collette had the capacity to make decisions about her continued relationship with Roisin.

Following their conversations with the Manager, and with support from the Dementia Specialist, the family decided not to visit the home at the same time as Roisin.

Some staff recognized that the relationship was a long standing and supportive one and were concerned about the attitude of the family. However, some staff continued to find this relationship between two females difficult to accept or comprehend.

Additional training on sexuality and intimacy was offered to all the staff in the Home. This helped the staff who had reservations about the relationship to understand their own feelings and enable them to be supportive of the relationship.

(Health and Social Care Board, 2020, pp.4–5)

This example shows how to keep the patient's best interests at the centre of all decision-making and how training can help staff to become more supportive. In such situations, it is important to seek guidance from regulatory bodies, adult protection agencies, and, where necessary, legal experts.

LGBTQ+ people with dementia who need advocacy and/or legal representation

Problems with families can become especially complex in relation to trans people with dementia. Indeed, it is the fear of many trans people that their families will influence care homes into recognizing the sex they were assigned at birth, and not the gender with which they now identify (Westwood & Price, 2016). In the US, some trans people who have died have been buried in the gender they did not identify with at the time of death, because their families of origin, who did not accept that they had transitioned, had arranged their funerals (Advocate, 2014). Sometimes trans people with dementia are pressured by their families of origin to conform to gender norms in ways which are at conflict with how they identify. It is important that staff and managers speak up on behalf of the person concerned.

The rights of LGBTQ+ people with dementia should always be upheld. It may be necessary to seek legal representation for them, and to consult with regulatory bodies, to ensure that those individuals who may have lost mental capacity have someone to advocate on their behalf. This person should be sensitive to LGBTQ+ issues and willing to advocate for the person with dementia to receive care and support that affirms their identifies and rights.

Conclusion

This chapter has highlighted the importance of speaking up for LGBTQ+ rights, on the small and big issues. Being assertive, and being able to constructively challenge, is essential. Sometimes it is necessary to draw the line with individuals who are speaking or behaving inappropriately about or towards LGBTQ+ people. It is important that the line is drawn clearly and carefully, leaving people with options. Making a care organization's values and standards clear from the outset plays an important role in setting the tone.

Some problems can be dealt with in-house. Sometimes expert advice, including legal advice, will need to be obtained. Always, always, someone must be empowering the person with dementia, ensuring that their voice is heard and that they are being advocated for if/when they are unable to advocate on their own behalf.

FOOD FOR THOUGHT

- Do you have a clear values statement? Is it on display? Do you make service users and visitors aware of it?

- Do you have a statement on how to handle abusive behaviour by visitors? Are all staff and visitors aware of it? Are all staff confident in how to apply it, and that they will be backed up by managers in doing so?

- How confident are staff and managers about being assertive in difficult situations? Can they all constructively challenge people and situations? Do they need support in developing their skills in this area?

- Do you have a strategy with how to deal with racist/sexist/homophobic/transphobic abuse by patients? If not, do you need to develop one? How? Who will lead on this?

- Do you have connections with organizations that can provide you with legal advice if needed?

- Do you have connections with adult protection agencies?

- Do you provide an advocacy service for all people with dementia?

KEY LEARNING POINTS

- ✓ Prevention is better than cure, and it is always better to create a culture that is LGBTQ+-inclusive before problems emerge.

- ✓ Problems can still arise, even when your organization is fully LGBTQ+-inclusive.

- ✓ Knowing how to challenge others is an important skill for life as well as work.

✓ Being able to challenge others is essential where part of your responsibility is to protect those who cannot defend themselves, and to uphold their rights.

✓ The important thing about challenging someone is that you focus on what it is they have said or done, not who they are.

✓ People can and do change, and challenging their behaviour can be part of their change process.

✓ Sometimes, LGBTQ+ people with dementia need advocacy. It is important that you speak up on their behalf, but also that you know who to turn to when issues are complex and there are competing interests involved.

Chapter 5

Summing Up and Next Steps

Chapter summary

This chapter:

✓ provides a *quick recap* of the previous chapters

✓ addresses three important issues which have cut across the chapters:

  — *Treating everyone as individuals*

  — *LGBTQ+ personhood and dementia care*

  — Understanding and *respecting LGBTQ+ families of choice*

✓ invites you to *reflect on your own attitudes towards LGBTQ+ people* and delivering care to them

✓ offers some *words of encouragement* for the way forward and invites you to identify the next steps you might wish to take

✓ signposts you to the *list of resources provided at the end of this book.*

Introduction

This final chapter first provides a quick recap of the previous chapters, before going on to consider four key themes which cut across all of the chapters. The first of these themes is about treating everyone as an individual. The second is about personhood in LGBTQ+ dementia care. The third is about LGBTQ+ families of choice. The fourth is about self-reflection. At the end of the chapter, we encourage you to think about your next steps in developing LGBTQ+-inclusive practice and services for people living with dementia, and signpost you to additional resources.

Quick recap

In Chapter 1, we explained why a good practice guide about LGBTQ+ people affected by dementia is necessary. We are not all the same, and we need not to be treated as all the same. Having a minority sexuality and/or gender identity, especially among current generations of older LGBTQ+ people, informs who and how we are, and how we feel about needing care. Sadly, much of dementia care provision is not yet geared up to meet the needs of LGBTQ+ people, and there can still be prejudice and discrimination in some places. Also, in Chapter 1, we gave a potted history of LGBTQ+ rights in the UK across recent decades, to help you put things in a wider context and understand some of the things older LGBTQ+ people in particular have gone through.

> I have cared for individuals in different care settings, who have been very guarded regarding their sexuality and gender identification, only since moving into the care home. These individuals had been very well known in the community but were afraid to be themselves within the care setting in case people treated them differently, which was extremely sad. *Natalie Lamoon, manager of Alexander House care home in Dover* (Learner, 2019, online)

Chapter 2 looked at how to deliver effective care to LGBTQ+ people. We explored the importance of recognizing, understanding, respecting and meeting the specific needs of LGBTQ+ people living with dementia. We explained how sometimes you have to treat people differently in order to treat them equally well.

All of the social care providers sell themselves as being LGBT inclusive, but few have any awareness of what that might look like in practice. There are good reasons why trans people say they will commit suicide rather than end up in social care. Professor Stephen Whittle (a trans man) (Whittle, 2020, p.12)

In Chapter 3, we discussed the 'safe space' approach – how to make people feel they can be open about themselves, welcomed and accepted. We explored LGBTQ+-inclusive policies and procedures and highlighted the importance of making sure that LGBTQ+ colleagues feel safe to be out at work. We addressed staff recruitment, training and development, LGBTQ+ community involvement in all aspects of a service, and LGBTQ+ carer support. We also gave an example of a care home which learned from its mistakes, which is all any of us can do.

There is thought to be around a million people over the age of 55 who identify as LGBT+, yet a new poll shows a lot more needs to be done to make care homes inclusive, with over a third of staff having had no LGBT awareness training. In the same survey, they found one in ten staff had witnessed their LGBT+ residents experiencing prejudice...

Alice Wallace, director of Opening Doors London, said: 'Our own survey carried out as part of the Pride in Care quality standard has resulted in very similar findings. For example, a third of staff didn't think knowing a person was LGBT+ was at all relevant to providing personalized care and almost 10 per cent said they did not feel responsible for providing care and support to LGBT+ people and, most worryingly, while 15 per cent of care staff had heard people make negative or hostile remarks about LGBT+ people at work there was a lack of clarity of what to do in those situations.'

A spokesperson for carehome.co.uk said: 'We would like to see more care homes being actively inclusive and investing in specialist LGBT+ training for their staff so that everyone feels equally valued.' (Learner, 2019, online)

In Chapter 4, we looked at dealing with challenges, particularly in relation to staff who may not agree with creating an LGBTQ+-inclusive service, and in relation to religious and cultural tensions, and to family members of people with dementia who may be prejudiced towards LGBTQ+ people. We also explored how to support LGBTQ+ people with dementia who may need independent advocacy.

Cutting across these chapters were some common themes, which we will now consider in a little more detail.

Treating everyone as individuals

We started this book reflecting on our sense that many people feel that it is necessary to take something of a blanket approach when working with people living with dementia – that is to say, that everyone should be treated the same and that this would, by definition, mean that everyone is treated equally. It is hoped that what you have read will have persuaded you that the opposite should be true in practice and that treating everyone differently, whatever their needs, should ensure that they get the same quality of care. This notion, obviously, applies to any person but has, we have argued, a particular resonance when it comes to working with LGBTQ+ people.

There is good practice out there, as some of our examples have shown. And the fact that you are reading this book shows that there is an appetite to learn and grow and to deliver the best possible service to each person living with dementia, including each and every LGBTQ+ individual living with dementia.

GOOD PRACTICE EXAMPLE 5.1

Some care providers are leading the way in being truly inclusive. Belong care villages are part of this small minority of residential care settings which are celebrating diversity.

They are tackling prejudice head on by hosting LGBT+ reminiscence events, attending Pride marches and even holding their own Silver Pride.

Stacey McCann, chief operating officer of care provider Belong, which runs seven care villages in the north of England, says: 'Belong has made great strides in proactively embracing the LGBT+ community in recent years through events and initiatives, including hosting regular LGBT+ events for older people, such as Silver Rainbows reminiscence sessions and Crewe's first ever Silver Pride event. This extends to supporting residents to attend Pride events in the wider community.

'As a values-based organization, committed to equality and promoting diversity, Belong actively seeks to create environments that are counteractive to prejudice, and where people can be comfortable expressing who they are. Part of this involves communicating Belong's inclusive values widely, including with signage.'

Belong has also invested in specialist training for its staff. Ms McCann adds: 'Many people living in a care setting who identify as LGBT+ would have found it much more difficult to express who they were when growing up than they would today, and some may still find it difficult as a result. When moving into a care setting, some may have worries because of prejudice they experienced in the past. The training covers how to identify if people have such concerns and how to support them emotionally if they are.'

Jane Chadbond, aged 59, who lives at Belong Wigan, has been involved with some of these LGBT events. She says: 'I can't imagine living somewhere where I felt the need to hide who I am. On the contrary, I feel at home at Belong, I've never experienced any discrimination or prejudice, and other LGBT people in my life feel comfortable visiting, which is very important to me. I think this is partly due to the staff clearly expressing their commitment to equality and supporting LGBT people, including helping me to attend Pride events in Wigan and Manchester.'

(Learner, 2019, online)

Personhood and dementia care

Personhood is very important to dementia care. This is how a famous writer in the world of dementia, Tom Kitwood, defined 'personhood':

The standing or status bestowed by one human being by others, in the context of human relationship and social being. It implies recognition, respect and trust. (Kitwood, 1997, p.8)

Kitwood's theories have been extremely influential in the world of dementia (Mitchell & Agnelli, 2015). They also have a wider relevance and resonance for care provision, particularly in those contexts where people have to rely on others for many of their day-to-day needs. However we provide care, whoever that care is provided for and to, and wherever it is provided, it all happens in the context of people-to-people interactions. How we relate to others in our care is hugely important to the quality of that care.

Kitwood said that people with dementia are often perceived, and responded to, through a 'deficit model', that is, one which focuses wholly on what is wrong with them, what they cannot do. All types of dementia are thought about in medical terms as being a direct result of damage to the brain which results in the symptoms and experiences that we term 'dementia'. This medical model of dementia has, traditionally, governed the understanding, diagnosis, treatment and care of people living with dementia. Many people would argue that the medical model has been responsible for the 'deficit model' of people living with dementia. Interventions and treatment are arguably constructed from a perspective of 'body maintenance' where all that is necessary is to keep the person with dementia 'fed, watered and kept clean'.

Of course, we hope your own practice will not reflect this approach. We hope you will understand that dementia is a complex interaction between a person's physical, social and interpersonal relationships which combine with some of the changes in the brain. People are more than their dementia. LGBTQ+ people are more than their dementia.

PAUSE FOR THOUGHT

We invite you to think for a moment about your own personhood. In short, what is it about you that makes you 'you'?

- What is it about 'you' that would still be 'you' even if you had dementia?

- What would you want carers who didn't know you to be aware of about you in order to effectively provide you with care?

- Who are the people who are important to you who you would like to be involved and included in your care?

- Who are the people in your world who you would not like to be involved and included in your care?

- What are the things you would wish to be supported in continuing to do?

Our interactions with the people we care for and support in a professional capacity should be person-centred, that is, they should begin with the person themselves, whose needs should drive the ways in which care is planned, delivered and evaluated. So, a care plan should not just be a dry piece of institutional paperwork. Rather, it should reflect an empowering and proactive approach to supporting the person to maintain their skills and attributes and achieve the things they wish to achieve, and, of course, it should help support them with any particular challenges they may face.

> When I'm 75 and needing residential or nursing home care, I am not going back in the closet. I spent my life fighting to get out of the closet. I'm not going back into the closet. I want to be able to talk to you if you're sitting next to me about how sad I am because I've lost the man in my life. I don't want to have to talk in language that doesn't cause offence. I'm not going back there when I'm 75 just because there's no other service available. *Andrew, gay man, aged 57* (Price, 2010)

LGBTQ+ personhood and dementia care
So, what does personhood look like in practice? How do you know if you are validating and supporting a person's personhood? In

some senses, the answer to this is very simple – start from where the person is, focusing on the unique needs, circumstances and preferences of the person being supported. In some senses, if you get dementia care 'right' for members of the LGBTQ+ community (or any minority group, for that matter), you will be getting it right for everyone you care for because this will mean that you genuinely are working in a person-centred way, taking each person's strengths, needs, aspirations, desires and so on into account in your work with them.

> The potential exists for the provision of care and support to older LGBTQ+[1] people to become a 'litmus test' – an indicator for how well health and social care agencies engage with minority groups and deliver a non-discriminatory service. (Ward, Pugh & Price, 2010, p.26)

This book has been encouraging you to develop an awareness of your own competence, and that of your organization, to work in a person-centred way with LGBTQ+ people living with dementia. You may have come across the term 'cultural competence'. This is the ability to engage ethically with a range of people with diverse values, beliefs and behaviours and to make respectful and reflexive decisions which value people's personal, social, and cultural needs. However, some LGBTQ+ authors are uncomfortable talking about an LGBTQ+ culture or even cultures because LGBTQ+ people are all so very different and do not belong to a single 'culture' (Westwood, 2020).

> My name is Patrick. I'm originally from Barbados. And I am the youngest person in the UK to be diagnosed with frontal lobe atrophy, which is a form of dementia... When I was diagnosed, I felt alone and I did not know where to turn. Services didn't suit a young gay man with dementia. I didn't and still don't have a partner to support me. While mine and everyone's experience of dementia is unique, there can be many challenges [with dementia] that are specific to a

---

1   The original quote used the LGB acronym, however we have modified this to LGBTQ+ to promote greater inclusiveness.

person's sexual orientation or gender identity. (Alzheimer's Society, 2019, video)

LGBTQ+ people with dementia vary by age, sex, sexuality, gender identity, race, ethnicity, ability/disability, religion, education and income.

> There is...a world of difference between the woman who has spent most of her adult life as a wife and mother, coming to same-sex relationships later, perhaps in her 40s or 50s, and at a time when social attitudes to lesbianism were becoming less punitive, and the 'never married', childless, life-long lesbian...who has lived for much of her life in secrecy and fear. The latter is statistically likely to be the most in need of support services for old people, and yet she is the least visible. The challenge for providers of those services, then, is first to realize that she exists and then to provide a context in which she can thrive, whether she ever 'comes out' or not. (Traies, 2016, p.235)

While it can be useful to talk about 'LGBTQ+ people' as a sort of shorthand, for convenience, the risk is that differences between LGBTQ+ people, including those with dementia, get lost along the way (Westwood, 2020). Some older LGBTQ+ people's voices – and needs – may end up being recognized and understood less well than others. So we prefer not to talk about 'LGBTQ+ cultural competence', but rather 'LGBTQ+ knowledge and understanding' instead.

No two people are the same, including no two LGBTQ+ people. Person-centred care is all about this, and about meeting each individual's needs on their own terms. We recommend applying several key principles in working with LGBTQ+ personhood in dementia care.

- First, we would suggest practising a sense of **openness** and **sensitivity** towards other people – this comes from an awareness, acceptance, and validation of difference (in all its forms).

- Second, we would suggest that a **critical approach** to

practice is essential to enable you to develop a sense of confidence in your knowledge and understanding. This means asking questions (even if they are awkward and the answers are difficult to hear) and not taking accepted cultural norms and behaviours as the benchmarks for your own practice.

- Practice with a sense of **humility** – being open to new learning and suspending your taken-for-granted ideas, attitudes and approaches will enable you to fully appreciate other people's perspectives and their own, perhaps different, worldviews.

- Be prepared to encounter and engage with **uncertainty**. There is seldom one right answer or approach when dealing with complex human beings. Sometimes, situations can be confusing and unclear, but accepting that this is a natural part of engaging with other people can make difficult situations far easier to manage.

GOOD PRACTICE EXAMPLE 5.2

Janet (white, Jewish background, 84 years old) is a trans woman who has recently moved in to your care home. She transitioned late in life and was happy being open about her transgender status when she first arrived. The other residents have accepted her. However, in the last 12 months she has begun to show signs of dementia and now has trouble remembering who she is. Some mornings she will wake up insisting that she is a man called Simon and be very confused as to why she has only women's clothes and is being called Janet. Other days she still identifies as Janet and gets very upset with anyone who calls her Simon.

- What are the key concerns here?

- How would you initially proceed?

- What would you want to know?

- How would current policies in the care home support your initial response?

- Are there any policies missing and how might you take this forward?

Top tips:

- Respect Janet's choices and recognize that these may change from day-to-day.

- Janet may need some reminders about the things that are important to her and interest her – knowing a bit more about Janet's life history is important. Having a collection of important photographs from Janet's past may help Janet to make sense of what's going on.

- Explore ways that the home can provide a mix of women's and men's clothes in Janet's bedroom so she has some choices each day and can access these easily.

- Janet's loved ones may find this experience distressing and need to be consulted on how they wish to be involved in her care. Keep in mind that Janet's loved ones may include friends as well as family members. Speak to Janet first about whom the home should communicate with. Showing signs of dementia doesn't mean Janet does not have the capacity to make her own decisions.

- Update staff members involved in Janet's care and make sure staff have an opportunity to ask questions and discuss concerns they may have.

- Ensure the home provides gender neutral facilities and bathrooms for all residents and staff to access, regardless of their gender identity.

Care Under the Rainbow Case Studies (School for Policy Studies, University of Bristol and Diversity Trust, 2019, p.4)

Understanding and respecting
LGBTQ+ families of choice

> I'm not typical of older gay men I think because I've got loads of friends and I've got loads of women friends. I'm very close to my sister and my niece who lives [abroad], she's got three children and I adore her. She came and stayed a week with me, we had a wonderful time, totally open with her about everything... But my friends are my family, lovely close friends I've got...there's just such a closeness, a feeling of mutual support. Emotional support. Always there for one another. Very mutual, not at all one sided. Happy times...like my friend if he ever has to go to the hospital or anything like that, I'll go with him. *Jack, gay man, aged 66* (quoted in Westwood, 2016c, p.91)

As we have identified earlier in the book, one of the ways in which LGBTQ+ people's lives may differ from those of the majority population is in the context of family life and what 'family' means in both theory and practice. We have already talked about the importance of understanding the significance of 'family of choice' (i.e. those significant relationships which go beyond family of origin and biological ties) in the lives of LGBTQ+ people. In this concluding chapter, we would like to explain this a little more. Like many people, LGBTQ+ people have diverse relationship networks, both in terms of how large or small they are, and in terms of who makes up those networks. For some LGBTQ+ people, those networks may not include, or only include to a small extent, their families of origin.

> And there will also be those of us, a sizeable population, who didn't bring our families along with us. We became distanced. I mean they're maintained, our links with our biological families, but they're not our first port of call. We look to our friends I think. *Alice, lesbian, aged 60* (quoted in Westwood, 2016c, p.90)

While many LGBTQ+ people, including older people, have rich social networks, not all do. Some have experienced family rejection and/or may have mental health issues linked to lifelong prejudice and discrimination, which make it difficult to form and maintain relationships. Others may have lived very concealed lives.

> I've only got one really good friend now, and he's a married guy, his wife doesn't know. But it's got to be limited all the time... It's not having a network of friends that depresses me. *Les, gay man, aged 62* (quoted in Westwood, 2016c, p.90)

In LGBTQ+ communities, some friendships are much more than 'just good friends' and are more like family relationships. And, for some LGBTQ+ people, their friendships are more important to them than their relationships with their family of origin.

> That's what's so comfortable about our community here, [it's] that we get it, we don't have to do any explaining. And that's why that community is comfortable. And that's why our wider blood family isn't. It's not that we keep having to justify it, but it's just like my sister, it doesn't matter how many nice meals she puts on the table, and smiles, and all the rest of it, she doesn't truly believe that we're normal [laughs]. So, why should you be comfortable around somebody who thinks you're a pervert? Whereas with our [lesbian] family, we know we're normal. *Daphne, lesbian, aged 60* (Westwood, 2016c, p.90)

Many LGBTQ+ people find a sense of connection and belonging with one another that they cannot find with non-LGBTQ+ people.

> Having other trans-identified friends normalizes my own trans experience for me simply by providing contact with someone who is 'like me'... It makes me feel like less of a freak to have contact with other people who share my experience. *Transgender research participant* (quoted in Galupo *et al.*, 2014, p.205)

On the other hand, not all LGBTQ+ people have things in common, and their networks of support may not always involve all LGBTQ+ people, but rather sub-groups of LGBTQ+ people, especially among older people, for example older lesbians supporting each other, older gay men supporting each other, older transgender people supporting each other.

> For those who have transitioned, specifically those who have undergone surgeries, hormone replacement therapies, or who are living as a gender different from what they were sexed at birth – all of these experiences are unique in our culture and because the trans experience is also highly stigmatized or emphasized as different, exotic, and so on that I can talk about my feelings and thoughts about my body and my daily life with other trans people. And to some extent, I can't share this sort of 'mirroring' with cis people. *Transgender research participant* (quoted in Galupo *et al.*, 2014, p.207)

The other thing to remember is that although older lesbians and gay men are less likely to have children and grandchildren, some do, many having been heterosexually married earlier in their lives. And for many, their relationships with their children and grandchildren are very important.

> We've been together since 1987... We had our civil ceremony in 2008 and my granddaughters were ring bearers. My two boys came. And David's son Michael, he was his best man. My girlfriend ['she's like my sister, we've known each other since I was three'] was my best man and his son was his best man, as it were. *Andrew, gay man, aged 66* (quoted in Westwood, 2016c, p.90)

Lastly, while many heterosexual people remain in contact with, and are supportive towards, ex-partners, this is especially common among older LGBTQ+ people. Many people in same-sex couples remain very close to their ex-partners, even when they are in new relationships.

> Moira [lesbian, aged 75] explains the significance of ex-partners: 'It's kind of family, they're family.'

> Jennifer (aged 62) has been with her present partner for over 20 years and describes her previous partner as 'kind of like a third person in our relationship'.

Ian (aged 69) and Arthur (aged 60) are 'best friends' with their ex-partners, who are now partnered to one another.

(Westwood, 2016c, p.94)

Many older LGBTQ+ people provide – and receive – care and support from ex-partners, especially during times of illness.

May's ex-partner has cancer and now lives with her: 'She's not back as my partner, she's back as a friend in need.' (May, aged 64).

Violet and Moira cared for Moira's ex-partner in the final years of her life ('There she is on our windowsill,' said Violet, aged 73, pointing to a photograph).

Des' ex-partner comes to stay with him in his sheltered accommodation... 'He stays in the guest suite on the ground floor.' (Des, aged 69).

(Westwood, 2016c, p.94)

While some people will, no doubt, have limited family and social networks, the social and familial networks of LGBTQ+ people may be far wider than you might, at first, imagine. There may be a network of potential support for the person living with dementia and for you in your professional capacity. If you are not able, or willing, to explore beyond the boundaries of what we traditionally understand as 'family', then you will be doing the person you're helping to support, and yourself, a profound disservice. Moreover, you will be denying yourself the opportunity to benefit from the knowledge and expertise of those people who may know the person you are caring for better than anyone else does.

Joan, aged 67: Maureen's ex-husband is painting the outside of our house.

Maureen, aged 62: [It's become amicable] It took a long time. We were OK with each other after a while, although it was a bit strained. But then he got ill. And I used to just pop in, have a quick coffee with him. He's fine now, he's OK.

Joan, aged 67: But he brings his problems to you...

Maureen, aged 62: Yes, he does, and the dog... He tried to get me to iron his shirt yesterday. He said 'You haven't ironed a shirt of mine for twenty years'. And I said 'I'm not starting now'. [Laughter]

Maureen and Joan, long-term lesbian couple
(quoted in Westwood, 2016c, p.95)

Self-reflection

Self-reflection is essential for everyone delivering care services to other people. As we explained at the beginning of this chapter, care delivery involves relationships, and respect for personhood. That involves respecting the person to whom you are delivering services. And by respect we don't mean simply tolerating or putting up with someone. We mean accepting the whole person, appreciating them, valuing them, and being interested in every aspect of who they are. It means celebrating their lives, whether they are lives like yours, or lives that are very different from yours. It means empathizing with the ways in which some people with dementia have experienced stressful lives in the past, and how some of those stressful experiences may inform how they perceive and receive your care.

BEING A REFLECTIVE PRACTITIONER

Reflection is the thought process where individuals consider their experiences to gain insights about their whole practice. Reflection supports individuals to continually improve the way they work or the quality of care they give to people. It is a familiar, continuous and routine part of the work of health and care professionals.

Opportunities for multi-professional teams to reflect and discuss openly and honestly what has happened when things go wrong should be encouraged. These valuable reflective experiences help to build resilience, improve wellbeing and deepen professional commitment. (Joint statement of support from Chief Executives of statutory regulators of health and care professionals [UK], Health and Care Professionals Council, 2019)

For LGBTQ+ people living with dementia, especially older LGBTQ+ people, 'minority stress' – i.e. the effects of prejudice and discrimination across their lives – has led to them to experience poorer physical and mental health, especially anxiety and depression. Some of that minority stress has resulted from prejudice and discrimination by health and social care providers, and this, understandably, makes older LGBTQ+ people very wary of engaging with those services when they need to in later life, including when they have dementia.

So, it is vital that services for people with dementia make sure that they are wholly LGBTQ+-inclusive. And an essential part of this is ensuring that each individual working directly with LGBTQ+ people with dementia is ready and able to be inclusive. They key question for you to reflect on is whether you feel ready and able to care for an LGBTQ+ person with dementia, and whether you think your team and your organization are too.

We really need to challenge our prejudices and reflect on our discriminatory views before we can go out and practice effectively. *Social worker* (Westwood, 2022c, p.11)

Dementia can be frightening, confusing, disorientating. It involves a loss of control of our lives and ourselves. And it involves a loss of privacy. Our lives go on show for all to see. And it is that loss of privacy that is so worrying for LGBTQ+ people, especially older LGBTQ+ people, because being able to shut their front doors and leave the world outside has often been the only way they have been able to feel safe. With dementia, that is lost. Not just for the person with dementia, but for their partners and close family and friends too.

As a care provider, stepping into the private worlds of LGBTQ+ people with dementia, it is important that you treat those worlds with dignity and respect. While we do not all find everyone easy to work with, finding a whole group of individuals difficult to work with, not because of personalities or dementia symptoms, but because of *who they are*, is a big problem. Now, many of you will not have a problem with working with LGBTQ+ people, be that colleagues or the people to whom you deliver services. Many of you may have friends or family members who identify with the LGBTQ+ community. Many of you will identify as LGBTQ+ yourselves. But for some of you, you may feel uncomfortable working with LGBTQ+ people. Some of you may come from cultural or religious backgrounds where LGBTQ+ people are disapproved of. Some of you may feel that if you just show compassion to LGBTQ+ people even though you disapprove of them or their 'lifestyles', that will be enough. It will not. Unless you can regard LGBTQ+ people's lives as having equal worth and rights as your own, you cannot deliver LGBTQ+-inclusive care. It is impossible to celebrate the lives of people you disapprove of. And it is impossible to challenge the discrimination they experience if you secretly believe it is justified.

OVERCOMING OUR OWN PREJUDICES

- Try to catch yourself judging someone.

- Ask yourself what proof you have that your judgment is based on truth.

- Challenge your judgments. Look for evidence that refutes your negative opinion of others.

- Remind yourself often that you:

  - might be mistaken in your judgment

  - cannot read minds

  - would be upset to think someone is judging you unfairly.

- Broaden your group of friends to include people you previously might have ignored.

- Remain alert to the influence of subtle stereotyping and other potential seeds of prejudice in TV, books, conversations, etc.

(Stewart, 2011, online)

We all have 'internalized homophobia' and 'internalized transphobia', that is, prejudiced thoughts and ideas about LGBTQ+ people that we have absorbed from the social messages and cues we have picked up across our lives. It is not the internalized prejudice that matters so much as what you do about it. If you deny it, and do not look at it, then it has power over you. If you look at it, examine it, question it for what it is, and make informed choices about how to act, knowing it is there, then you take back your power. It does not control you.

> We really need to challenge our prejudices and reflect on our discriminatory views before we can go out and practice effectively. *Social worker* (Westwood, 2022c, p.11)

So, we would ask each and every one of you to examine your internalized homophobia and internalized transphobia, without guilt or shame, and with self-compassion and understanding. It is not your fault! What is your responsibility is what you do about it and how you go forward in your life, and in your work, once you know that it is there.

It is important to self-reflect all the time. At the end of a shift, a working day, a working week, pause and allow yourself to think about all that you have said and done, what you are pleased with, what you think you could have done better, what you have learned from this, and how you will do better in the future. We are all works in process, and that includes our approach to delivering care and support to LGBTQ+ people affected by dementia.

Final words

We hope this book has given you the confidence to perhaps revisit some of your taken-for-granted assumptions and understandings of the lives of older LGBTQ+ people and, in particular, those people who have a diagnosis of dementia. The issue of sexuality and/or gender identity is a thread that weaves through LGBTQ+ people's journeys through dementia, and this point of profound vulnerability is precisely where LGBTQ+ people are in need of informed understanding and validation. To conclude, we would like to challenge you and your organization to ensure that you provide that understanding and advocacy using, we hope, this book to help inform your own, and each other's, future practice.

Next steps

In terms of next steps, you may want to do several things. First, think about how, as an individual, you feel about working with LGBTQ+ people with dementia, and whether there is anything you need to address in order to work positively with them, their families and friends. Second, identify any training needs you think you might have. And third, go and get those training needs met.

Managers and organizational leaders may also wish to conduct an audit of your care services' policies and procedures, ascertaining whether your LGBTQ+ staff feel confident and supported in the workplace, and your staff's attitudes towards, and knowledge and understanding of the needs and concerns of LGBTQ+ people with dementia. Having got to this point in the book, you may have some ideas about what other sorts of things you could explore in such an audit with a view to making your services fully LGBTQ+-inclusive.

Even simply asking yourself and your colleagues questions about practice in this context could be very revealing in identifying people's values and elements of good, and less positive, practice. No doubt some people would say, 'Why do we need a special audit for LGBTQ+ people? Why is dementia different for them?' But, we hope, having read this book, you will now be able to give a very well-informed answer to those questions.

We have also provided a list of sources of further information, guidance and support at the end of this book. But also, do reach out to LGBTQ+ organizations in your local area. Many will be delighted to collaborate with you. There is no better way to find out about LGBTQ+ people's needs than talking with LGBTQ+ people themselves. Don't be afraid to ask.

FOOD FOR THOUGHT

- Try writing your own care plan, imagining that you have a diagnosis of dementia. Some of the questions that you might want to consider are: What is your biography? Which people are important to you? What particular difficulties might you have and what are the key things that would help you to manage these challenges. What sort of things may distress you and how can you be best supported with this? What are your needs for dignity and privacy? Obviously, your care plan will differ markedly from that of other people precisely because you are a unique individual, as is every other person requiring professional care and support. Whatever your physical (arguably basic) needs might be, however, we would guess that, for most people, the things that are most important to them and what they would want professionals to know most about them would be the nature and quality of their relationships with other people.

- Based on what you have read in this book, what do you think might be some of the things that could be important to a lesbian, or a gay man, or a bisexual woman or man, or a transgender person who is living with dementia that they might want to put in their care plans? Do you think relationships will also be at the heart of them?

- Given that relationships are all important to dementia care, and that dementia care goes beyond 'feeding, watering and keeping clean', how important is it that people providing care to LGBTQ+ people with dementia should feel positively towards them? Can someone learn to feel positive about LGBTQ+ people?

KEY LEARNING POINTS

✓ Treating each person as an individual is essential for respecting their personhood.

✓ Relationships are all-important, especially the relationships we build with the people in our care, and we must be sure to respect and validate those relationships.

✓ For some LGBTQ+ people with dementia, their significant relationships may take different forms from those people with dementia who do not identify as LGBTQ+.

✓ It is essential to recognize, respect and include those individuals and relationships which are significant for an LGBTQ+ person with dementia in their care.

✓ Self-reflection is vital to monitor, and learn from, your attitudes towards LGBTQ+ people and the ways in which you deliver their care.

Glossary

BIPHOBIA	Prejudice and discrimination towards bisexual people.
CISGENDER	Women and men who identify with their biological sex.
CIS	An abbreviation for cisgender (e.g. cis woman, cis man).
CROSS-DRESSER	'Someone who wears the clothes usually expected to be worn by someone of the "opposite" gender. Other terms include "transvestite" (now becoming a dated term and disliked by some) and "dual role". A cross-dresser is unlikely to have a full-time identity as a member of their cross-dressed gender and typically does not seek medical intervention' (Government Equalities Office and Gendered Intelligence, 2015, p.19).
GENDER	Cultural and social constructions of femininity and masculinity.
GENDER IDENTITY	The gender(s) with which one identifies.
HETERONORMATIVE	The assumption that heterosexuality is the normal way of being.
HETEROSEXISM	The privileging of heterosexuality.
HOMOPHOBIA	Prejudice and discrimination towards lesbian, gay and bisexual people.
INTERSEX	People born with a reproductive anatomy that does not fit the binary categories of male or female (this is extremely rare).
LGB	Lesbian, gay and bisexual.
LGBT	Lesbian, gay, bisexual and transgender.
LGBTQ	Lesbian, gay, bisexual, transgender and queer.

LGBTQ+	'…lesbian, gay, bisexual, transgender, queer (or sometimes questioning), and others. The "plus" represents other sexual identities including pansexual' (Cherry, 2022).
	'Other acronym variations that are sometimes used include LGBTQIA+ (lesbian, gay, bisexual, transgender, queer, intersex, asexual, plus other identities), LGBTIQ (lesbian, gay, bisexual, transgender, intersex and queer), and LGBTQQIP2SAA (lesbian, gay, bisexual, transgender, queer, questioning, intersex, pansexual, two-spirit (2S), androgynous, and asexual)' (Cherry, 2022).
QUEER	'Queer is a term used by those wanting to reject specific labels of romantic orientation, sexual orientation and/or gender identity. It can also be a way of rejecting the perceived norms of the LGBT community (racism, sizeism, ableism etc.). Although some LGBT people view the word as a slur, it was reclaimed in the late 80s by the queer community who have embraced it' (Stonewall 2020c).
SEX	The observable biological differences between male, female and intersex people.
SEXUAL IDENTITY	The sexual identity with which one identifies, among those who understand sexuality in terms of identity, for example lesbian, gay, bisexual, heterosexual, pansexual.
SEXUAL ORIENTATION	The gendering of sexual desire, based on which gender(s) one finds sexually attractive/desirable, among those who understand sexuality in terms of orientation – orientated to 'same', 'different', 'both' or multiple gender/sexes.
SEXUALITY	Encompasses sexual identity, sexual orientation, sexual performance and sexual desires.
TRANS	Describes people who are transgender, and those who do not identify with the gender binary (i.e. neither male or female). This includes people who are 'transsexual, gender-queer (GQ), gender-fluid, non-binary, gender-variant, crossdresser, genderless, agender, nongender, third gender, bi-gender…and neutrois' (Stonewall, 2020c).

TRANSGENDER	Transgender people do not identify with their biological sex at birth. Transgender women (trans woman/trans women) were born as biological males but identify as female. Transgender men (trans man/trans men) were born as biological females but identify as male.
TRANSITION	To undergo a process (or part of a process) by which a person changes their physical sex characteristics and/or gender expression to match their inner sense of being male or female (or other). This process may include a name change, a change in preferred pronouns, and a change in social gender expression through things such as hair, clothing and mannerisms. It may or may not include hormones and surgery (adapted from Lambda Legal 2013, p.1).
TRANSPHOBIA	Prejudice and discrimination towards transgender people.
TRANSSEXUAL	A transgender woman or man who is transitioning/has transitioned.

References

Advocate (2014) Outrage After Idaho Trans Woman Buried 'As a Man', 24 November. www.advocate.com/politics/transgender/2014/11/24/outrage-after-idaho-trans-woman-buried-man

Age UK (2011) *Transgender issues in later life*. London: Age UK.

Age UK (2017) *Safe to be me: Meeting the needs of older lesbian, gay, bisexual and transgender people using health and social care services*. London, Age UK. www.ageuk.org.uk/globalassets/age-uk/documents/booklets/safe_to_be_me.pdf

Alabaster, G. (2022) *Top 10 tips for LGBT inclusion in the workplace*. Stonewall. www.stonewall.org.uk/about-us/news/top-10-tips-lgbt-inclusion-workplace

Almack, K. (2018) 'I Didn't Come Out to Go Back in the Closet': Ageing and End of Life Care for Older LGBT People. In A. King, K. Almack, Y.T. Suen & S. Westwood (eds), *Older Lesbian, Gay, Bisexual and Trans People: Minding the Knowledge* Gaps. Abingdon: Routledge.

Alzheimer's Association and SAGE Advocacy Services for LGBT Elders. (Undated) *Issues Brief: LGBT and Dementia*. www.lgbtagingcenter.org/resources/pdfs/lgbt-dementia-issues-brief.pdf

Alzheimer's Society (2019) *What is 'Bring Dementia Out'?* (video). www.youtube.com/watch?v=io6600RFDbU

Anchor (2022) *Our Culture and Values*. www.anchor.org.uk/careers/why-join-us/our-culture-and-values

Baker, C. & Maegusuku-Hewett, T. (2011) *Dignified social care with transgender older people: A literature review*. Swansea University: https://cronfa.swan.ac.uk/Record/cronfa13830/Details

Baril, A. & Silverman, M. (2019) Forgotten lives: Trans older adults living with dementia at the intersection of cisgenderism, ableism/cogniticism and ageism. *Sexualities*, 25(1–2). https://doi.org/10.1177/1363460719876835

Barnes, D., Boland, B., Linhart, K. & Wilson, K. (2017) Personalisation and social care assessment–the Care Act 2014. *British Journal of Psychiatry Bulletin*, 41(3), 176–180.

Barrett, C., Crameri, P., Lambourne, S., Latham, J.R. & Whyte, C. (2015) Understanding the experiences and needs of lesbian, gay, bisexual and trans Australians living with dementia, and their partners. *Australasian Journal on Ageing*, 34, 34–38.

Barrett, C., Crameri, P., Latham, J. R., Whyte, C. & Lambourne, S. (2016) Person-Centred Care and Cultural safety. In S. Westwood & E. Price (eds), *Lesbian, Gay, Bisexual and Trans* Individuals Living with Dementia: Concepts, Practice and Rights*, pp.97–109. Abingdon: Routledge.

Being Me Project (2020) *Best practice principles on developing LGBT cultural competence in health and social care education*. Amersfoort, The Netherlands. https://beingme.eu/public/application/downloads/resources/being-me-best-practice-principles-20200622.pdf

Birch, H. (2009) *Dementia, lesbians and gay men*. Alzheimer's Australia. https://dhs.sa.gov.au/__data/assets/pdf_file/0017/74150/Dementia,-lesbians-and-gay-men.pdf

Bouman, W.P., Claes, L., Marshall, E., Pinner, G.T. *et al.* (2016) Sociodemographic variables, clinical features, and the role of preassessment cross-sex hormones in older trans people. *The Journal of Sexual Medicine*, 13(4), 711–719.

Bristowe, K., Marshall, S. & Harding, R. (2016) The bereavement experiences of lesbian, gay, bisexual and/or trans* people who have lost a partner: A systematic review, thematic synthesis and modelling of the literature. *Palliative Medicine*, 30(8), 730–744.

Cant, B. & Hemmings, S. (eds) (2010) *Radical Records (Routledge Revivals): Thirty Years of Lesbian and Gay History, 1957–1987*. London: Routledge.

Carr, S. & Ross, P. (2013) *Assessing current and future housing and support options for older LGB people*. York: Joseph Rowntree Foundation. www.jrf.org.uk/file/43285/download?token=yQXrwM09&filetype=summary

Care Quality Commission (CQC) (2019) *Relationships and sexuality in adult social care services: Guidance for CQC inspection staff and registered adult social care providers*. www.cqc.org.uk/sites/default/files/20190221-Relationships-and-sexuality-in-social-care-PUBLICATION.pdf

Care Quality Commission (CQC) (2022) *Equality and human rights*. www.cqc.org.uk/about-us/our-strategy-plans/equality-human-rights

Cherry, N. (2022) *What Does LGBTQ+ Mean? Understand Why the Acronym is Used and What It Stands for*. Very Well Mind (Online), 18 July. www.verywellmind.com/what-does-lgbtq-mean-5069804

Concannon, L. (2009) Developing inclusive health and social care policies for older LGBT citizens. *British Journal of Social Work*, 39(3), 403–417.

Correro, A.N. & Nielson, K.A. (2020) A review of minority stress as a risk factor for cognitive decline in lesbian, gay, bisexual, and transgender (LGBT) elders. *Journal of Gay & Lesbian Mental Health*, 24(1), 2–19.

Cousins, E., De Vries, K. & Dening, K.H. (2021) LGBTQ+ people living with dementia: An under-served population. *British Journal of Healthcare Assistants*, 15(1), 26–35.

Crameri, P., Barrett, C., Lambourne, S. & Latham, J.R. (2015) *We are still gay: An evidence based resource exploring the experiences and needs of Lesbian, Gay, Bisexual and Trans Australians living with dementia*. www.dementia.org.au/sites/default/files/NATIONAL/documents/Dementia-Narrative-Resource.pdf

Dementia Support (2022) LGBT Dementia Support. www.dementiasupport.org.uk/news/lgbt-dementia-support

Department of Health and Social Care (DHSC) (2021) *Care and support statutory guidance*. August 2021. London: DHSC.

Di Lorito *et al.* (2021) Are dementia services and support organizations meeting the needs of Lesbian, Gay, Bisexual and Transgender (LGBT) caregivers of LGBT people living with dementia? A scoping review of the literature. *Aging and Mental Health*, 26(10), 1912–1921. https://doi.org/10.1080/13607863.2021.2008870

DiPlacido, J. (1998) *Minority Stress Among Lesbians, Gay Men, and Bisexuals: A Consequence of Heterosexism, Homophobia, and Stigmatization.* New York, NY: Sage Publications.

Equality and Human Rights Commission (2011) Close to home: An inquiry into older people and human rights in home care. www.equalityhumanrights.com/en/publication-download/close-home-inquiry-older-people-and-human-rights-home-care

Fairbairn, C., Pyper, D. & Balogun, B. (2022) *Gender Recognition Act reform: Consultation and outcome.* London: House of Commons Library. https://researchbriefings.files.parliament.uk/documents/CBP-9079/CBP-9079.pdf

Fish, J. (2006) *Heterosexism in Health and Social Care.* London: Springer.

FORGE (2011) Quick Tips for Caregivers of Transgender Clients. https://forge-forward.org/resource/quick-tips-for-caregivers-of-transgender-clients

Fredriksen-Goldsen, K.I., Cook-Daniels, L., Kim, H.J., Erosheva, E.A *et al.* (2014) Physical and mental health of transgender older adults: An at-risk and underserved population. *The Gerontologist*, 54(3), 488–500.

Galupo, M.P., Bauerband, L.A., Gonzalez, K.A., Hagen, D.B., Hether, S.D. & Krum, T.E. (2014) Transgender friendship experiences: Benefits and barriers of friendships across gender identity and sexual orientation. *Feminism & Psychology*, 24(2), 193–215.

Gay & Lesbian Health Victoria (GLHV), (2016) *LGBTI-Inclusive Practice Audit Tool for Health and Human Service Organizations* (second edition). La Trobe University, Australia: GLHV. https://rainbowhealthaustralia.org.au/media/pages/research-resources/lgbti-inclusive-practice-audit-tool/3547223994-1650953507/lgbti-inclusive-practice-audit-tool.pdf

Godfrey, C. (2018) Section 28 protesters 30 years on: 'We were arrested and put in a cell up by Big Ben'. *The Guardian* [Online] 27 March. www.the-guardian.com/world/2018/mar/27/section-28-protesters-30-years-on-we-were-arrested-and-put-in-a-cell-up-by-big-ben

Government Equalities Office and Gendered Intelligence (2015) *Providing services for transgender customers: A guide.* London: Government Equalities Office. https://assets.publishing.service.gov.uk/government/uploads/system/uploads/attachment_data/file/484857/Providing_services_for_transgender_customers-a_guide.pdf

Guasp, A. (2011) *Lesbian, Gay and Bisexual People in Later Life.* London: Stonewall.

Hafford-Letchfield, T., Simpson, P., Willis, P.B. & Almack, K. (2018) Developing inclusive residential care for older lesbian, gay, bisexual and trans (LGBT) people: An evaluation of the care home challenge action research project. *Health & Social Care in the Community*, 26(2), e312–e320. https://doi.org/10.1111/hsc.12521

Hafford-Letchfield, T., Willis, P., Almack, K. & Simpson, P. (2016) Developing an LGB T&I inclusive environment for older people living in care homes: Community advisors assessment and development tool. Middlesex University, London in Association with Comic Relief. www.caremanagementmatters.co.uk/wp-content/uploads/2017/04/Community-Advisors-Assessment-and-Development-Tool.pdf

Health and Care Professions Council (2019) *Benefits of becoming a reflective practitioner. Joint statement of support from Chief Executives of statutory regulators of health and care professionals.* www.hcpc-uk.org/globalassets/news-and-events/benefits-of-becoming-a-reflective-practitioner----joint-statement-2019.pdf

Health and Social Care Board (2020) *Relationships, Sexuality and Dementia.* Northern Ireland Social Care Council. https://hscboard.hscni.net/relationships-sexuality-dementia

Healthwatch (2018) *Trans Health, Care & Wellbeing.* www.diversitytrust.org.uk/wp-content/uploads/2018/07/Healthwatch-Trans-Health-Care-and-Wellbeing-Report-03.04.18.pdf

Higgins, A., Downes, C., Sheaf, G., Bus, E. *et al.* (2019) Pedagogical principles and methods underpinning education of health and social care practitioners on experiences and needs of older LGBT+ people: Findings from a systematic review. *Nurse Education in Practice,* 40, 102625.

House of Commons Women and Equalities Committee (2019) *Health and Social Care and LGBT Communities. First Report of Session 2019.* HC 94. https://publications.parliament.uk/pa/cm201919/cmselect/cmwomeq/94/94.pdf

Hughes, M. & Robinson, P. (2019) Gay Men and Ageing. In S. Westwood (ed.), *Ageing, Diversity and Equality: Social Justice Perspectives,* p.114. Abingdon: Routledge.

Hunt, R., Cowan, K. & Chamberlain, B. (2007) *Being the gay one: Experiences of lesbian, gay and bisexual people working in the health and social care sector.* London: Stonewall. https://hscbusiness.hscni.net/pdf/DH-_LGBT_people_working_in_health_and_social_care_pdf.pdf

Hunter, C., Bishop, J.A. & Westwood, S. (2016) The Complexity of Trans*/Gender Identities: Implications For Dementia Care. In S. Westwood & E. Price (eds), *Lesbian, Gay, Bisexual and Trans* Individuals Living with Dementia* (pp.144–157). Abingdon: Routledge.

Jen, S. & Jones, R.L. (2019) Bisexual lives and aging in context: A cross-national comparison of the United Kingdom and the United States. *The International Journal of Aging and Human Development,* 89(1), 22–38.

Jones, R.L. (2016) Sexual Identity Labels and their Implications in Later Life: The Case of Bisexuality. In E. Peel & R. Harding (eds), *Ageing and Sexualities: Interdisciplinary Perspectives.* Abingdon: Routledge.

Jones, R.L., Almack, K. & Scicluna, R.M. (2016) Ageing and bisexuality: Case studies from the Looking Both Ways project. Project report. Open University Press, Milton Keynes, UK.

Jones, R.L., Almack, K. & Scicluna, R. (2018) Older bisexual people: Implications for social work from the 'Looking Both Ways' study. *Journal of Gerontological Social Work,* 61(3), 334–347.

Jones, S.M. & Willis, P. (2016) Are you delivering trans positive care? *Quality in Ageing and Older Adults,* 17(1), 50–60.

Jones-Schenk, J. (2018) Creating LGBTQ-inclusive care and work environments. *The Journal of Continuing Education in Nursing*, 49(4), 151–153.

King's College London ACCESSCare Research (2017) *Palliative and end-of-life care for LGBT people.* https://www.ncbi.nlm.nih.gov/pmc/articles/PMC5758934

Kitwood T. (1997) *Dementia Reconsidered: The Person Comes First.* Buckingham: Open University Press.

Knocker, S. (2006) *The Whole of Me: Meeting the Needs of Older Lesbians, Gay Men and Bisexuals Living in Care Homes and Extra Care Housing. A Resource Pack for Professionals.* London: Age Concern. http://docs.sciesocialcareonline.org.uk/fulltext/104375.pdf

Knocker, S. (2012) *Perspectives on Ageing: Lesbians, Gay Men and Bisexuals.* London: Joseph Rowntree Foundation.

Lambda Legal (2013) *Creating Equal Access to Quality Health Care for Transgender Patients: Transgender-Affirming Hospital Policies.* www.lambdalegal.org/publications/fs_transgender-affirming-hospital-policies

Learner, S. (2019) *Back in the closet: Third of care home staff have had no LGBT+ awareness training.* www.carehome.co.uk/news/article.cfm/id/1611092/back-closet-third-care-home-staff-no-lgbt-training

LGBT Age (2015) *Creating a safe space.* www.lgbthealth.org.uk/wp-content/uploads/2015/01/Creating-a-safe-space.pdf

LGBT Health and Wellbeing (2014) *Ten Top Tips: A guide for services and organizations working with older people for becoming more inclusive of lesbian, gay, bisexual and transgender people.* www.lgbthealth.org.uk/wp-content/uploads/2014/07/Top-Ten-Tips.pdf

LGBT Health and Wellbeing (2020) *Proud to Care: LGBT and Dementia.* www.lgbthealth.org.uk/wp-content/uploads/2021/06/LGBT-Dementia-Toolkit-2020.pdf

Lim, F., Jones, P.A. & Paguirigan, M. (2019) A guide to fostering an LGBTQ-inclusive workplace. *Nursing Management*, 50(6), 46–53.

Löf, J. & Olaison, A. (2020) 'I don't want to go back into the closet just because I need care': Recognition of older LGBTQ adults in relation to future care needs. *European Journal of Social Work*, 23(2), 253–264.

Manthorpe, J. & Samsi, K. (2016) Person-centered dementia care: Current perspectives. *Clinical Interventions in Aging*, 11, 1733.n

Marie Curie (2017) *Hiding Who I Am: The Reality of End-of-Life Care for LGBT People.* London: Marie Curie. www.mariecurie.org.uk/globalassets/media/documents/policy/policy-publications/hiding-who-i-am-the-reality-of-end-of-life-care-for-lgbt-people.pdf

Marie Curie (2020) *Getting care and planning for the future. Information for LGBTQ+ people affected by terminal illness, and their family and friends*: www.eel.nhs.uk/sites/default/files/lgbtq-booklet-getting-care-and-planning-for-the-future.pdf

McGovern, J. (2014) The forgotten: Dementia and the aging LGBT community. *Journal of Gerontological Social Work*, 57(8), 845–857.

McParland, J. & Camic, P.M. (2018) How do lesbian and gay people experience dementia? *Dementia*, 17(4), 452–477.

Miles, N. (2011) *Straight Allies: How they help create gay-friendly workplaces.* www.equality.admin.cam.ac.uk/files/straight_allies.pdf

Mitchell, G. & Agnelli, J. (2015) Person-centred care for people with dementia: Kitwood reconsidered. *Nursing Standard*, 30(7), 46–50.

Musingarimi, P. (2008) *Social Care Issues Affecting Older Gay, Lesbian and Bisexual People in the UK: A Policy Brief.* London: The International Longevity Centre (ILCUK).

National Care Forum (UK) (2016) *Dementia and LGBT Communities.* www. nationalcareforum.org.uk/wp-content/uploads/2019/10/Dementia-care-and-LGBT-communities.pdf

National Housing Federation (2022) Anchor Hanover/Older LGBT+ people's needs. www.housing.org.uk/our-work/diversity-and-equality/case-studies/anchor-hanover--older-lgbt-peoples-needs

National LGBT Center (2013) *Affirmative Care for Transgender and Gender Non-Conforming People: Best Practices for Front-line Health Care Staff.* Boston, MA: Fenway Institute.

NHS National End of Life Care Programme (2012) *The route to success in end of life care – achieving quality for lesbian, gay, bisexual and transgender people.* www.macmillan.org.uk/documents/aboutus/health_professionals/endoflifecare-lgbtroutetosuccess.pdf

Nowaskie, D.Z. & Sewell, D.D. (2021) Assessing the LGBT cultural competency of dementia care providers. *Alzheimer's & Dementia: Translational Research & Clinical Interventions*, 7(1), e12137.

Peel, E. & McDaid, S. (2015) *'Over the Rainbow': Lesbian, Gay, Bisexual, Trans People and Dementia Project. Summary Report.* http://eprints.worc.ac.uk/3745/1/Over-the-Rainbow-LGBTDementia-Report.pdf

Power, L. (1995) *No Bath But Plenty of Bubbles: An Oral History of the Gay Liberation Front, 1970–1973.* London: Cassell.

Price, E. (2008) Pride or prejudice? Gay men, lesbians and dementia. *British Journal of Social Work*, 38(7), 1337–1352.

Price, E. (2010) Coming out to care: Gay and lesbian carers' experiences of dementia services. *Health & Social Care in the Community*, 18(2), 160–168.

Psychology Today (2022) *Assertiveness.* www.psychologytoday.com/gb/basics/assertiveness#:~:text=Assertiveness%20is%20a%20social%20skill,positions%2C%20and%20boundaries%20to%20others

Pugh, S. (2012) Care Anticipated: Older Lesbians and Gay Men Consider Their Future Needs. In R. Ward, I. Rivers & M. Sutherland (eds), *Lesbian, Gay, Bisexual and Transgender Ageing: Biographical Approaches for Inclusive Care and Support* (pp.41–54). London: Jessica Kingsley Publishers.

Riggs, D.W. & Kentlyn, S. (2014) Transgender Women, Parenting, and Experiences of Ageing. In M. Gibson (ed.), *Queering Motherhood: Narrative and Theoretical Perspectives* (pp.221–232) Toronto: Demeter Press.

Rosenfeld, D., Bartlam, B. & Smith, R.D. (2012) Out of the closet and into the trenches: Gay male baby boomers, aging, and HIV/AIDS. *The Gerontologist*, 52(2), 255–264.

Royal College of Nursing (RCN) (2016) *Caring for lesbian, gay, bisexual or trans clients or patients: Guide for nurses and health care support workers on next of kin issues.* London: RCN. www.rcn.org.uk/Professional-Development/publications/pub-005592

School for Policy Studies, University of Bristol and Diversity Trust (2019) *Care Under the Rainbow Case Studies.* www.diversitytrust.org.uk/careunderrainbow

Sharpe, A.N. (2007) Endless sex: The Gender Recognition Act 2004 and the persistence of a legal category. *Feminist Legal Studies*, 15(1), 57–84.

Simpson, P. (2013). Alienation, ambivalence, agency: Middle-aged gay men and ageism in Manchester's gay village. *Sexualities*, 16(3–4), 283–299.

Simpson, P., Almack, K. & Walthery, P. (2018) 'We treat them all the same': The attitudes, knowledge and practices of staff concerning old/er lesbian, gay, bisexual and trans residents in care homes. *Ageing & Society*, 38(5), 869–899.

Skills for Care (2020) *Equality and diversity*. www.skillsforcare.org.uk/Developing-your-workforce/Care-topics/Equality-and-diversity/Equality-and-diversity.aspx

Social Care Institute for Excellence (2011) '*Working with lesbian, gay, bisexual and transgender people: older people and residential care: Roger's story.' Transcript of video*. www.scie.org.uk/lgbtqi/video-stories/older-people-residential-care

Social Care Institute for Excellence (2020) *LGBT+ communities and dementia*. www.scie.org.uk/dementia/living-with-dementia/lgbt

Spiegelhalter, D. (2015) Is 10% of the population really gay? *The Guardian* [Online] 5 April. www.theguardian.com/society/2015/apr/05/10-per-cent-population-gay-alfred-kinsey-statistics

Stewart, L. (2011) Perhaps you work hard to resist prejudice, but do you have subtler forms of it in your thoughts? Online blog, *Solutions*, 12 December. www.valueoptions.com/solutions/2011/12-December/story5.htm

Stonewall (2015) *Unhealthy Attitudes*. www.stonewall.org.uk/resources/unhealthy-attitudes-2015

Stonewall (2020a) *What's the UK's LGBT population?* www.stonewall.org.uk/help-advice/faqs-and-glossary/student-frequently-asked-questions-faqs

Stonewall (2020b) *What's the UK's trans population?* www.stonewall.org.uk/help-advice/faqs-and-glossary/student-frequently-asked-questions-faqs

Stonewall (2020c) *Glossary of Terms*. www.stonewall.org.uk/help-advice/faqs-and-glossary/glossary-terms

Suffolk Lesbian, Gay, Bisexual and Transgender Network (2012) *Providing quality care to LGBT+ clients with dementia in Suffolk: a guide for practitioners*. www.lgbtagingcenter.org/resources/pdfs/providingLGBTclientcare.pdf

Sumerau, J.E., Barbee, H., Mathers, L.A. & Eaton, V. (2018) Exploring the experiences of heterosexual and asexual transgender people. *Social Sciences*, 7(9), 162.

Switchboard (2018) LGBTQ+ Communities & Dementia Engagement Report. www.switchboard.org.uk/wp-content/uploads/2018/09/LGBTQ-Dementia-Report_Final.pdf

Trades Union Congress (TUC) (2019) *How to be a good trans ally at work*. www.tuc.org.uk/sites/default/files/2019-11/Trans_Ally_Guidance_2019.pdf

Traies, J. (2015) Old lesbians in the UK: Community and friendship. *Journal of Lesbian Studies*, 19(1), 35–49.

Traies, J. (2016) *The Lives of Older Lesbians: Sexuality, Identity & the Life Course*. London: Springer.

Traies, J. (ed.) (2018) *Now You See Me: Lesbian Life Stories*. Wales: Tollington Press.

Walker, R., Hughes, C., Ives, D. & Jardine, Y. (2013) *Assessment of care needs and the delivery of care to older lesbians living in residential care homes in Bradford and Calderdale*. Bradford: The Labrys Trust.

Ward, R., Pugh, S. & Price, E. (2010) *Don't look back?: Improving health and social care service delivery for older LGB users*. Manchester: Equality and Human Rights Commission.

Watt, N. (2009) David Cameron apologises to gay people for section 28. *The Guardian* [Online] 2 July. www.theguardian.com/politics/2009/jul/02/david-cameron-gay-pride-apology

Weston, K. (1997) *Families We Choose: Lesbians, Gays, Kinship*. New York, NY: Columbia University Press.

Westwood, S. (2016a) 'We see it as being heterosexualised, being put into a care home': Gender, sexuality and housing/care preferences among older LGB individuals in the UK. *Health & Social Care in the Community*, 24(6), e155–e163.

Westwood, S. (2016b) Dementia, women and sexuality: How the intersection of ageing, gender and sexuality magnify dementia concerns among lesbian and bisexual women. *Dementia*, 15(6), 1494–1514.

Westwood, S. (2016c) *Ageing, Gender and Sexuality: Equality in Later Life*. Abingdon: Routledge.

Westwood, S. (2017a) Gender and older LGBT* housing discourse: The marginalised voices of older lesbians, gay and bisexual women. *Housing, Care and Support*, 20(3), 100–109.

Westwood, S. (2017b) Religion, sexuality, and (in) equality in the lives of older lesbian, gay, and bisexual people in the United Kingdom. *Journal of Religion, Spirituality & Aging*, 29(1), 47–69.

Westwood, S. (2020) The myth of 'older LGBT+' people: Research shortcomings and policy/practice implications for health/care provision. *Journal of Aging Studies*, 55, https://doi.org/10.1016/j.jaging.2020.100880

Westwood, S. (2022a) Religious-based negative attitudes towards LGBTQ people among healthcare, social care and social work students and professionals: A review of the international literature. *Health and Social Care in the Community*. https://doi.org/10.1111/hsc.13812

Westwood, S. (2022b) 'People with faith-based objections might display homophobic behaviour or transphobic behaviour': Older LGBTQ people fears about religious organizations and staff providing long-term care. *Journal of Religion, Spirituality & Aging*, http://dx.doi.org/10.1080/15528030.2022.2070820

Westwood, S. (2022c) Can religious social workers practice affirmatively with LGBTQ service recipients? An exploration within the regulatory context. *Journal of Social Welfare and Family Law*, 44(2), 205–225. www.tandfonline.com/doi/pdf/10.1080/09649069.2022.2067652

Westwood, S., Hafford-Letchfield, T. & Toze, M. (2021a) *The impact of COVID-19 on the lives of older lesbians in the UK*. University of York, University of Strathclyde & University of Lincoln: https://covid19olderlgbt.wordpress.com/155-2

Westwood, S., Hafford-Letchfield, T. & Toze, M. (2021b) *The impact of COVID-19 on the lives of older gay men in the UK.* University of York, University of Strathclyde & University of Lincoln: https://covid19olderlgbt.wordpress.com/155-2

Westwood, S., James, J. & Hafford-Letchfield, T. (in press) 'He's a gay, he's going to Hell'–Negative nurse attitudes towards LGBTQ people on a UK hospital ward: A single case study analysed in regulatory contexts. *Ethics and Social Welfare.*

Westwood, S., King, A., Almack, K. & Suen, Y-T (2015) Good Practice in Health and Social Care Provision for Older LGBT People. In J. Fish & K. Karban (eds), *Social Work and Lesbian, Gay, Bisexual and Trans Health Inequalities: International Perspectives*, pp.145–159. Bristol: Policy Press.

Westwood, S. & Knocker, S. (2016) One-Day Training Courses on LGBT* Awareness – Are they the Answer? In S. Westwood & E. Price (eds), *Lesbian, Gay, Bisexual and Trans* Individuals Living with Dementia: Concepts, Practice and Rights* (pp.155–167). Abingdon: Routledge.

Westwood, S. & Price, E. (2016) *Lesbian, Gay, Bisexual and Trans* Individuals Living with Dementia: Concept, Practice, and Rights.* Abingdon: Routledge.

Whittle, S. (2020) Written evidence submitted by Stephen Whittle [GRA2010] https://committees.parliament.uk/writtenevidence/18336/pdf

Willis, P., Raithby, M., Dobbs, C., Evans, E. & Bishop, J.A. (2020) 'I'm going to live my life for me': Trans ageing, care, and older trans and gender non-conforming adults' expectations of and concerns for later life. *Ageing & Society*, 41(12), 2792–2813. doi:10.1017/S0144686X20000604

Witten, T.M. (2016) Trans* People Anticipating Dementia Care. In S. Westwood & E. Price (eds), *Lesbian, Gay, Bisexual and Trans* Individuals Living with Dementia* (pp.110–123). Abingdon: Routledge.

World Health Organization (2022) Dementia: Key Facts. www.who.int/news-room/fact-sheets/detail/dementia

Useful Contacts and Resources

Contacts
UK
NATIONAL LGBT ORGANIZATIONS

LGBT Consortium: www.consortium.lgbt

LGBT Foundation (Manchester): http://lgbt.foundation

LGBT Health and Wellbeing (Scotland): www.lgbthealth.org.uk

Opening Doors (London): www.openingdoorslondon.org.uk

Rainbow Project (N. Ireland): www.rainbow-project.org

Switchboard (Brighton and Hove): http://switchboard.org.uk

Stonewall Cymru (Wales): www.stonewallcymru.org.uk

Stonewall Scotland: www.stonewallscotland.org.uk

Stonewall (UK): www.stonewall.org.uk

Stonewall Housing: https://stonewallhousing.org

DEMENTIA ORGANIZATIONS

Alzheimer's Society: www.alzheimers.org.uk

Alzheimer Scotland: www.alzscot.org

Alzheimer's Society Cymru (Wales): www.alzheimers.org.uk/about-us/wales

Alzheimer's Society Northern Ireland: www.alzheimers.org.uk/about-us/alzheimers-society-northern-ireland

Dementia UK: www.dementiauk.org

US

NATIONAL LGBT ORGANIZATIONS
GLAAD: www.glaad.org

Lambda Legal: www.lambdalegal.org

The National Resource Center on LGBTQ+ Aging: www.lgbtagingcenter.org

Old Lesbians Organizing for Change (OLOC): https://oloc.org

DEMENTIA ORGANIZATIONS
Alzheimer's Association: www.alz.org

Dementia Friends USA: https://dementiafriendsusa.org

National Council of Certified Dementia Practitioners: www.nccdp.org

Canada

NATIONAL LGBT ORGANIZATIONS
Advocacy Canada LGBT: https://advocacy-canada.lgbt

Egale Canada Human Rights Trust: https://egale.ca/about

DEMENTIA ORGANIZATIONS
Alzheimer Society of Canada: https://alzheimer.ca/en

Australia

NATIONAL LGBT ORGANIZATIONS
LGBTQI+ Health Australia: www.lgbtiqhealth.org.au

DEMENTIA ORGANIZATIONS
Dementia Australia: www.dementia.org.au

Resources
Written materials

- *Affirmative Care for Transgender and Gender Non-Conforming People: Best Practices for Front-line Health Care Staff* (USA): www.lgbtqiahealtheducation.org/publication/affirmative-services-for-transgender-and-gender-diverse-people-best-practices-for-frontline-health-care-staff

- *Dementia, lesbians and gay men* (Australia): https://dhs.sa.gov.au/__data/assets/pdf_file/0017/74150/Dementia,-lesbians-and-gay-men.pdf

- *Getting care and planning for the future Information for LGBTQ+ people affected by terminal illness, and their family and friends* (UK): www.eel.nhs.uk/sites/default/files/lgbtq-booklet-getting-care-and-planning-for-the-future.pdf

- *LGBTI and Dementia: Understanding changes in behaviour* – free booklet (Australia): www.lgbtiqhealth.org.au/lgbti_and_dementia_understanding_changes_in_behaviour_resource

- *LGBTI-inclusive practice audit tool for health and human service organizations. 2nd edition* (Australia): https://rainbowhealthaustralia.org.au/media/pages/research-resources/lgbti-inclusive-practice-audit-tool/3547223994-1650953507/lgbti-inclusive-practice-audit-tool.pdf

- *Safe to be me: Meeting the needs of older lesbian, gay, bisexual and transgender people using health and social care services* (UK): www.ageuk.org.uk/globalassets/age-uk/documents/booklets/safe_to_be_me.pdf

- *We Are Still Gay: An evidence based resource exploring the experiences and needs of Lesbian, Gay, Bisexual and Trans Australians living with dementia* (Australia): www.dementia.org.au/sites/default/files/NATIONAL/documents/Dementia-Narrative-Resource.pdf

- *Proud to Care: LGBT and Dementia* (UK): www.lgbthealth.

org.uk/wp-content/uploads/2021/06/LGBT-Dementia-Toolkit-2020.pdf

- *Providing quality care to LGBT+ clients with dementia in Suffolk: a guide for practitioners* (UK): www.lgbtagingcenter.org/resources/pdfs/providingLGBTclientcare.pdf

- *Quick Tips for Caregivers of Transgender Clients*: https://forge-forward.org/resource/quick-tips-for-caregivers-of-transgender-clients

- *Ten Top Tips: A guide for services and organizations working with older people for becoming more inclusive of lesbian, gay, bisexual and transgender people* (UK): www.lgbthealth.org.uk/wp-content/uploads/2014/07/Top-Ten-Tips.pdf

- *Working with older lesbian, gay and bisexual people A Guide for Care and Support Services* (UK): www.stonewall.org.uk/system/files/older_people_final_lo_res.pdf

Videos

- *Bring Dementia Out* (Alzheimer's Society UK): www.youtube.com/watch?v=io66ooRFDbU

- *Edie: a day in the life of a lesbian with younger onset dementia* (Val's LGBTI Ageing & Aged Care, Australia): www.youtube.com/watch?v=LGFUQhCkT6U

- *LGBTI People and Dementia – Mary and Thelma* (Alzheimer's Australia SA): www.youtube.com/watch?v=PXreqt9elwI

- *LGBTI People and Dementia – Tony and Paul* (Alzheimer's Australia SA): www.youtube.com/watch?v=GhsicqAt-gY

- *Working with LGBT people – older people and residential care: Roger's story* (SCIE, UK): www.youtube.com/watch?v=8JRckToRgP4

- *LGBTI People and Dementia – Desi* [trans woman] (Alzheimer's Australia SA): www.youtube.com/watch?v=6If_Ff-qcfE

LGBTQ+ AGEING

- *Gen Silent* (US), free trailer: www.youtube.com/watch?v=fV3O8qz6Y5g

- *LGBT Seniors Tell Their Stories* (LA LGBT Center, USA): www.youtube.com/watch?v=JDOdv792rBA

- *LGBTI: Inclusion and Awareness in the aged care* (Australian Government Department of Health): www.youtube.com/watch?v=TvpXe_gDv1E

- *Never Too Late To Come Out As Transgender: Heartfelt Stories* (TRACS, UK): www.youtube.com/watch?v=vMAiJr4OZyI

- *Not Another Second: LGBT+ seniors share their stories* (Watermark Retirement Communities, USA): www.youtube.com/watch?v=q43kBuC_ups

- *Now You See Me: a film about a group of Older Lesbians* (Esme Waldron, UK): www.youtube.com/watch?v=T1sSewj4yMw

- *Opening Doors London* (UK): www.youtube.com/watch?v=JpKSRU90oyo

- *Then and Now – Older Lesbians Share Their Stories* (Val's LGBTI Ageing & Aged Care, Australia): www.youtube.com/watch?v=1IRUzuU6ZgE

- *Then and Now – Older Trans Women Share Their Stories* (Val's LGBTI Ageing & Aged Care, Australia): www.youtube.com/watch?v=92GOtFyFNrs

- *Then and Now – Trans Men Share Their Stories* (Val's LGBTI Ageing & Aged Care, Australia): www.youtube.com/watch?v=OOmVptpKQUA

- *Too Old to Remember: song of stories of LGBT older people* (Sally Goldsmith, UK): www.youtube.com/watch?v=yhwfbk5eMLs

Index